The I

Drug Therapy
and Breastfeeding

From Theory to Clinical Practice

Drug Therapy and Breastfeeding

From Theory to Clinical Practice

Thomas W. Hale, RPh PhD

Department of Pediatrics,
Texas Tech University School of Medicine Amarillo, Texas, USA

Kenneth F. Ilett, BPharm PhD

Department of Pharmacology,
University of Western Australia, Crawley, Western Australia, Australia

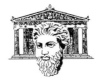

The Parthenon Publishing Group
International Publishers in Medicine, Science & Technology

A CRC PRESS COMPANY

BOCA RATON   LONDON   NEW YORK   WASHINGTON, D.C.

Published in the USA by
The Parthenon Publishing Group
345 Park Avenue South, 10th Floor
New York, NY 10010, USA

Published in the UK and Europe by
The Parthenon Publishing Group
23–25 Blades Court
London, SW15 2NU, UK

Library of Congress Cataloging-in-Publication Data

Data available on request from publisher

British Library Cataloguing-in-Publication Data

Hale, Thomas W.
   Drug therapy and breastfeeding : from theory to clinical practice
   1.Breast feeding 2.Drugs - Side effects 3.Drugs - Prescribing
   I.Title II.Ilett, Kenneth F.
   613.2'69

   ISBN 1-84214-110-4

Printed and bound by Bookcraft (Bath) Ltd., Midsomer Norton, UK

Contents

Preface

It is now well known that breastfeeding is the finest immunization a mother can give to her infant and produces major reductions in infectious and other diseases. Accordingly, worldwide interest in breastfeeding has increased, and progressively more mothers are choosing to breastfeed their infants. With this heightened interest, the need to know about the use of medications in breastfeeding mothers and the implications of this use for their infants have grown rapidly.

Assessing the safety of breastfeeding during maternal drug therapy requires an individual risk–benefit analysis that includes consideration of the amount of medication transferred to the infant via milk each day, the bioavailability of the drug to the infant, the age of the infant, and the potential adverse effects of the medication on the infant. It is generally agreed that many of the medications that are used in the perinatal period are relatively safe for breastfeeding mothers, and several books, reviews, and even the US Academy of Pediatrics provide lists of hazardous and safe medications.

The objectives of this book are to give the reader an understanding of mechanisms of drug transfer into human milk, to summarize current knowledge of infant dose and safety for major drug groups, and to provide a set of tools for evaluating the safe use of all medications that may be used during breastfeeding.

Thomas W. Hale
and **Kenneth F. Ilett**

Chapter 1

Introduction

1.1 Benefits of breastfeeding

Breastfeeding has very significant benefits for both mothers and their infants (for a recent review see Howard and Lawrence[1]). Infants benefit from an optimal nutritional diet and protection against infection because of antimicrobial, immune-stimulating and anti-inflammatory factors in the milk[2-4]. Breastfeeding also protects the infant against the development of food allergies, sudden infant death syndrome and diseases such as insulin-dependent diabetes mellitus, cardiovascular disease and ulcerative colitis[5-8]. Benefits to breastfeeding women include less postpartum blood loss, prompt uterine involution, more desirable inter-pregnancy intervals, and a lower lifetime risk of breast and ovarian cancer. Finally there is enhanced mother–infant bonding and maternal self-esteem. Given these benefits, it is not at all surprising that healthcare providers and mothers need information that would enable informed risk–benefit decisions to be made about drug use during lactation.

1.2 Alveolar subunit

A full description of the anatomy of the breast and physiology of lactation can be found in the text by Lawrence and Lawrence[9]. The parenchyma of the breast consists of approximately 10–15 ducts extending from the nipple and terminating in grape-like clusters termed alveoli. Each alveolus is lined with secretory cells called alveolar epithelial cells which are ultimately responsible for milk production (Figure 1.1). During pregnancy the size and number of alveolar complexes increase, although the high levels of maternal estrogen and progestogens inhibit actual milk production by suppressing alveolar epithelial cell function. Following delivery of the placenta, the rapid decrease of progestogen levels activates the alveolar cells and milk production ensues. In this early postpartum period, the milk produced is called colostrum and contains high concentrations of immunoglobulins and lactoferrin. Maternal plasma cells such as lymphocytes and macrophages are also transferred into milk, particularly in the early postpartum period when the alveolar epithelium is poorly developed. With each ensuing hour, the alveolar cells enlarge in size and the once-open intercellular gaps begin to disappear. After approximately 36–48 h, milk content enters its 'mature' stage, when maternal components such as sodium and chloride can no longer readily pass from the interstitial spaces into the lumen of the mammary alveoli[11]. The alveolus is surrounded by a rich supply of capillaries, which significantly increase in number during pregnancy. The surface of the alveolus is enveloped with a specialized smooth

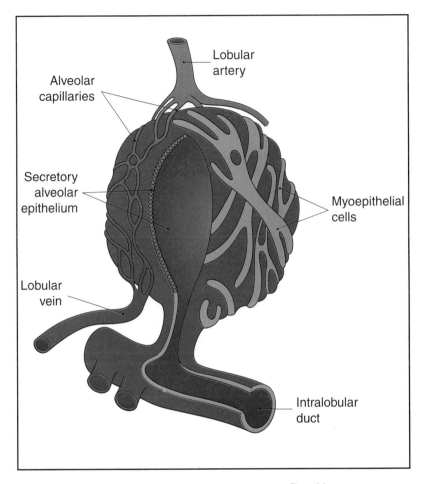

Figure 1.1
Typical mammary alveolus with contractile myoepithelial cells arrayed on the surface along with vasculature and intralobular ducts. The secretory alveolar epithelium lines the interior of the alveolar apparatus. Adapted and modified from reference 10

muscle cell called the myoepithelial cell. Nipple stimulation together with release of oxytocin from the mother's pituitary induces the myoepithelial cells to contract and force milk out toward the nipple (the 'letdown process').

1.3 Drug distribution into human milk

The transfer of drugs into human milk is usually facilitated by passive diffusion and the overall rate and extent of transfer may be affected by the stage of alveolar development, physicochemical characteristics of the drug (pKa, lipid solubility, relative molecular mass), the patient (drug concentration in the plasma) or the milk (aqueous, lipid and protein content). These mechanisms have been reviewed previously[12,13] with the most influential factors being as follows:

- Concentration of drug in the maternal plasma
- Plasma protein binding in the maternal plasma
- Fat content of milk – highly lipid soluble drugs show increased transfer in hind-milk compared with fore-milk
- Milk pH – milk is 0.2 pH units less than plasma and may lead to 'ion trapping' of some drugs
- Relative molecular mass of the drug – only small molecules (< 200–300 Da) penetrate readily

Early postpartum, with an underdeveloped alveolar epithelium, the transfer of drugs into human milk is higher than later, with mature milk. With large gaps existing between alveolar cells (Figure 1.2), drugs

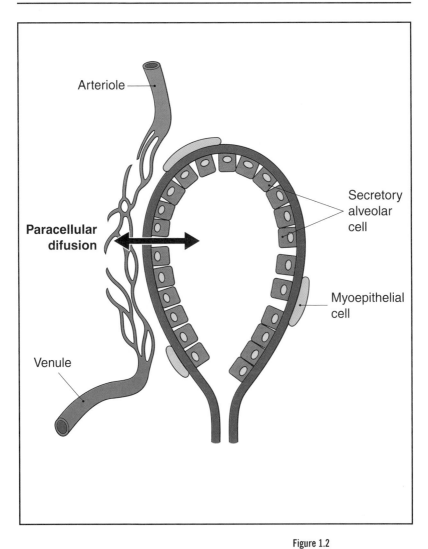

Arteriole

Paracellular
difusion

Venule

Secretory
alveolar
cell

Myoepithelial
cell

Figure 1.2
Model alveolus illustrating smaller
alveolar cells early postpartum
with large intercellular gaps, thus
permitting transfer of macrophages, lymphocytes and other
maternal substances

present in interstitial fluids can easily transfer directly into the milk by a process of aqueous diffusion. This is called the 'paracellular' pathway. While the overall drug concentration in milk may be high owing to the low volume of colostrum secreted, the absolute dose of drug transferred is probably low. Nevertheless, drug use in this early period should be approached cautiously. With growth of the alveolar epithelium, the intercellular gaps close and drugs must then transfer into milk by diffusion through the lipid membranes of the alveolar cells (Figure 1.3). For most drugs, transfer into and out of the alveolar cell is accomplished mainly by passive diffusion (Figure 1.4). This is called the 'transcellular' pathway. Once inside the alveolar cell, some lipid soluble drugs may also dissolve in the milk fat droplets and be co-secreted into the alveolar milk, thus enhancing their concentration in the milk. The paracellular pathway for aqueous diffusion of drugs into the milk through the gap junctions in the immature alveolar epithelium is probably significant only very early postpartum, as these junctions are closed by 48–72 h after birth.

Milk and plasma can be considered as two separate physiologic compartments in the breastfeeding mother (Figure 1.5). The mother may clear drugs in part by metabolism, and the nursing infant may therefore be exposed to both the parent drug and/or its metabolites. In turn, the infant ingests the drug orally and drug concentration (and effect) are controlled by oral absorption, as well as hepatic and renal clearance mechanisms. For the most part, the drug may transfer between milk and plasma in

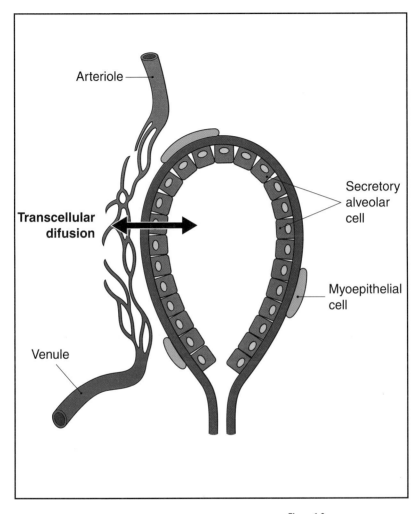

Arteriole

Transcellular difusion

Venule

Secretory alveolar cell

Myoepithelial cell

Figure 1.3
Model alveolus illustrating enlarged alveolar cells later postpartum (> 48 h) with minimal intercellular gaps, thus reducing transfer of larger maternal proteins, many medications, and maternal plasma cells

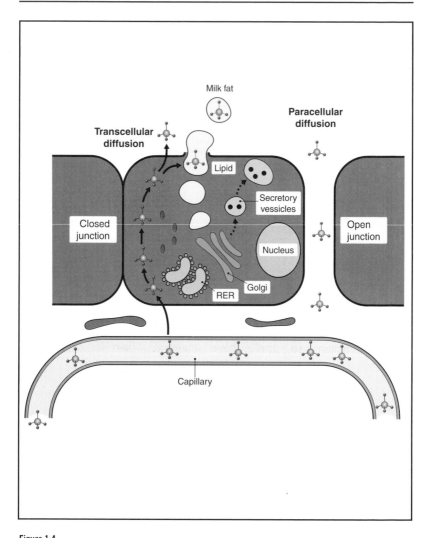

Figure 1.4

Secretion of milk components by the alveolar epithelium and passage of drugs into and out of the alveolar epithelial cell. Modified from reference 14. RER, rough endoplasmic reticulum

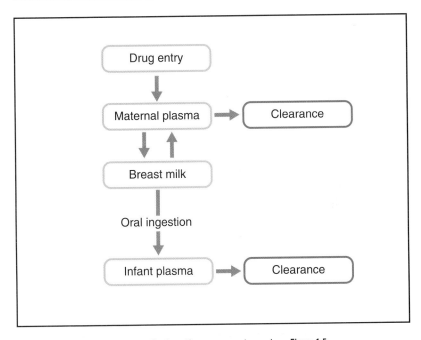

either direction so that these maternal compartments are in equilibrium most of the time, particularly during chronic therapy. This is illustrated for the antidepressant fluoxetine and its active metabolite norfluoxetine in Figure 1.6. For these drugs, milk and plasma concentration-time profiles are approximately parallel with 0.7:1 and 0.6:1 distribution ratios (between milk and plasma) for fluoxetine and norfluoxetine respectively.

The ratio of the concentration of drug in the milk to that in the plasma is known as the milk:plasma (M/P) ratio. While M/P is useful in understanding why drugs may penetrate into the milk, there are practical difficulties in measuring it accurately[16] as it may change from one hour to the next. In addition, M/P is of no direct use in assessing the likelihood

Figure 1.5
Compartmental representation of drug distribution in maternal plasma and milk and transfer to the suckling infant

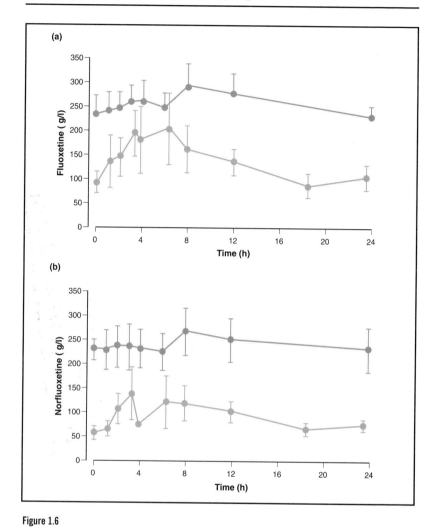

Figure 1.6

Plasma (●) and milk (●) concentration-time profiles for fluoxetine (a) and norfluoxetine (b) in 4 volunteers over a dose interval at steady-state. All data are corrected to the median daily dose of 40 mg fluoxetine and are presented as mean ± s.e.m. Some negative error bars have been omitted for clarity. Adapted with permission from Blackwell Science Publishers, Oxford, UK from Kristensen JH, Ilett KF, Hackett LP, *et al*. Distribution and excretion of fluoxetine and norfluoxetine in human milk. *Br J Clin Pharmacol* 1999;48:521–7

that a particular drug is safe to use during breastfeeding. Ultimately, it is the concentration of drug in the milk (C_{milk}) that determines infant exposure and enables safety to be assessed. Indirectly, M/P can sometimes assist in calculating milk drug concentration when only maternal plasma concentration is known:

$$C_{milk} = C_{plasma} \times M/P$$

Because of individual differences in the rate of transfer, the concentration–time profile of drug in the milk does not always parallel that in the plasma[17]. Thus, peak plasma concentrations (C_{max}) from the literature will not always be a reliable predictor of the likely time of peak in the milk. Actual measurements of drug concentrations in milk over a dose interval are therefore the best way to get reliable estimates of C_{max} and average concentration (C_{av}). Moreover, these concentrations can be used to estimate maximum or average infant exposure to the drug respectively.

M/P may exhibit significant between-sample variability. This is illustrated for the drug bupropion, used for smoking cessation and as an antidepressant, in Figure 1.7. The plasma and milk profiles measured[18] in a patient taking 100 mg three times daily were not parallel, and M/P varied from 2.4 to 8.5 over the dose interval. However, a more robust and informative M/P of 4.4 can be calculated as the ratio of the areas under the milk and plasma concentration–time curves respectively. Variability in single-point M/P values may arise from analytic variation, but is more often controlled by the

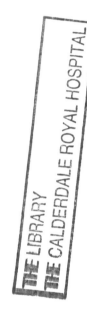

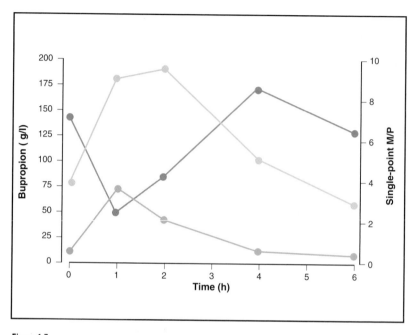

Figure 1.7

Concentration of bupropion in plasma (●) and breast milk (○) and single-point M/P (●) following a 100 mg oral dose. Drawn from data provided in Briggs et al[18]. An M/P of 4.4 was calculated using the ratio of area under the milk and plasma concentration–time curves respectively

physicochemical properties of the drug itself. It is interesting to note that while M/P for bupropion was highly variable, the M/P values for its hydrophilic metabolites hydroxybupropion and threohydro-bupropion were highly reproducible. Hence, if M/P is to be measured, the use of AUC data is always preferred[19].

DRUG THERAPY AND BREASTFEEDING

References

1. Howard CR, Lawrence RA. Drugs and breastfeeding [Review]. *Clin Perinatol* 1999;26:447–78

2. Numazaki K, Asanuma H, Hotsubo T, *et al*. Anti-human cytomegalovirus effects of breast milk. *J Infect Dis* 1996;174:444–5

3. Goldman AS. The immune system of human milk: antimicrobial, antiinflammatory and immunomodulating properties. *Pediatr Infect Dis J* 1993;12:664–71

4. Goldman AS, Chheda S, Garofalo R, *et al*. Cytokines in human milk: properties and potential effects upon the mammary gland and the neonate. *J Mammary Gland Biol Neoplasia* 1996;1:251–8

5. Hirose K, Tajima K, Hamajima N, *et al*. A large-scale, hospital-based case-control study of risk factors of breast cancer according to menopausal status. *Jpn J Cancer Res* 1995;86:146–54

6. Virtanen SM, Rasanen L, Aro A, *et al*. Feeding in infancy and the risk of type 1 diabetes mellitus in Finnish children. The 'Childhood Diabetes in Finland' Study Group. *Diabetic Med* 1992;9:815–19

7. Brinton LA, Potischman NA, Swanson CA, *et al*. Breastfeeding and breast cancer risk. *Cancer Causes Control* 1995;6:199–208

8. Cunningham AS, Jelliffe DB, Jelliffe EF. Breast-feeding and health in the 1980s: a global epidemiologic review. *J Pediatr* 1991;118:659–66

9. Lawrence RA, Lawrence RM. *Breastfeeding*, 5th edn. St Louis: Mosby, 1999

10. Vorherr H. *The Breast: Morphology, Physiology, and Lactation*. New York: Academic Press, 1974

11. Neville MC, Allen JC, Archer PC, *et al*. Studies in human lactation: milk volume and nutrient composition during weaning and lactogenesis. *Am J Clin Nutr* 1991;54:81–92

12. Atkinson HC, Begg EJ. Prediction of drug distribution into human milk from physicochemical characteristics. *Clin Pharmacokinet* 1990;18:151–67

13. Anderson PO. Drug use during breast-feeding [Review]. *Clin Pharm* 1991;10:594–624

14. Neville MC. The physiological basis of milk secretion [Review]. *Ann NY Acad Sci* 1990;586:1–11

15. Kristensen JH, Ilett KF, Hackett LP, *et al*. Distribution and excretion of fluoxetine and norfluoxetine in human milk. *Br J Clin Pharmacol* 1999;48:521–7

16. Begg EJ, Atkinson HC. Modelling of the passage of drugs into milk [Review]. *Pharmacol Ther* 1993;59:301–10

17. Wojnar-Horton RE, Hackett LP, Yapp P, *et al*. Distribution and excretion of sumatriptan in human milk. *Br J Clin Pharmacol* 1996;41:217–21

18. Briggs GG, Samson JH, Ambrose PJ, *et al*. Excretion of bupropion in breast milk. *Ann Pharmacother* 1993;27:431–3

19. Atkinson HC, Begg EJ, Darlow BA. Drugs in human milk. Clinical pharmacokinetic considerations. *Clin Pharmacokinet* 1988;14:217–40

Chapter 2

Infant exposure to drugs

2.1 Drug concentration in the plasma

The concentration of drug in the infant's plasma (C_{inf}) is a function of the dose ingested in the milk (D_{inf}), the drug's bioavailability (F) and the infant's clearance (CL_{inf}):

$$C_{inf} = \frac{D_{inf} \times F}{CL_{inf}}$$

Both hepatic and renal clearance mechanisms in infants mature to adult levels or higher over weeks or months following birth[1]. Thus, drug CL is often lower and half-lives correspondingly longer, in infants than in adults. Begg has estimated infant CL to be 5, 10, 33, 50, 66 and 100% of adult maternal levels at 24–28, 28–34, 34–40, 40–44, 44–68 and > 68 weeks post-conceptual age respectively[2].

Since the infant's drug exposure is via the oral route, F may be important. Values of F in infants are rarely available, but in general one would anticipate low values for those drugs that are known to have high first-pass clearance, and low F in adults. Infant F would be expected to be highest at birth and to decrease as hepatic and intestinal enzymes mature.

2.2 Calculation of infant dose

The important parameter of infant dose (D_{inf}) can be calculated as follows, where C_{max} and C_{av} are the maximum and average drug concentrations in milk, respectively:

D_{inf} = Drug concentration in milk (C_{max} or C_{av}) × volume of milk ingested

The volume of milk ingested varies with the age of the infant[3] and the extent to which the infant is 'fully' breastfed. Where there is no supplementary feeding, an average value of 0.15 l/kg/day has been recommended for such calculations[4]. Normalization of the dose to body weight (e.g. mg or μg/kg/day) is then used to facilitate interpretation of exposure.

2.3 Interpreting infant exposure

The simplest method of considering the safety of estimated infant dose is to relate the weight-normalized dose to that used during drug therapy in infants, or in children or adults where specific infant data are not available. However, the most useful measure of exposure is to calculate the relative infant dose.

Relative infant dose = D_{inf} (mg/kg/day)/Maternal dose (mg/kg/day)

This value is often expressed as a percentage. It provides a standardized means of relating the infant exposure to the maternal exposure. However it should be noted that the calculation assumes that the maternal dose lies within the 'usual' range of therapeutic doses.

The above discussion highlights two important points. Firstly, for full-term and older infants, the permitted relative infant dose should always be conservative. Bennett[4] recommends that a relative infant dose value that is greater than 10% of the maternal dose should be the notional 'level of concern' when considering the acceptability of drug exposure.

Secondly, premature infants have even lower clearance capacity than their full-term counterparts, and the 10% 'level of concern' may need to be lowered appropriately. In this regard, it should always be remembered that many neonates may have been exposed *in utero* to drugs taken by their mothers and that this level of exposure may be an order of magnitude greater than that received via breast milk.

2.4 Example of infant dose calculation

The calculation of absolute and relative infant doses for the antidepressant paroxetine is illustrated in Table 2.1, using data from Stowe and colleagues[5] (Figure 2.1). Stowe and his collaborators measured maximum paroxetine concentrations in milk from women taking different daily doses of paroxetine and derived a line of best fit. Average maximum paroxetine concentrations (μg/l) read off this line

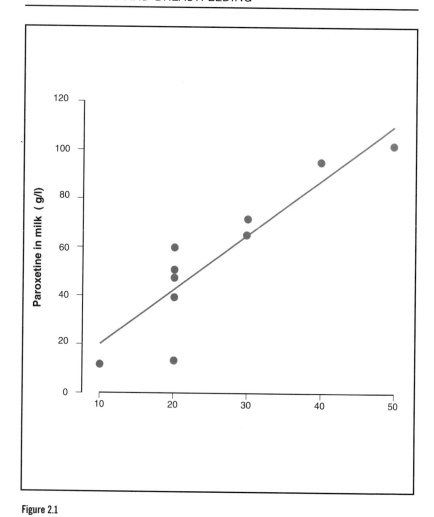

Figure 2.1

Maximum paroxetine concentrations (●) in human milk in a group of 10 women taking varying doses of paroxetine. The line of best fit is also shown. Redrawn after Stowe ZN, Cohen LS, Hostetter A, *et al*. Paroxetine in human breast milk and nursing infants. *Am J Psychiatry* 2000;157:185–9. ©2000 The American Psychiatric Association. Adapted and reproduced by permission

Table 2.1 Calculation of infant dose using paroxetine as an example

Maternal dose[a] (mg/d)	Paroxetine (μg/kg/d)	Paroxetine (μg/l, maximum)	Infant dose Absolute (μg/kg/d)	Infant dose Relative (%)
10	154	20	3.0	1.95
20	308	42	6.3	2.05
30	462	68	10.2	2.21
40	615	90	13.5	2.20
50	769	110	16.5	2.15

[a] Average body weight of 65 kg assumed

Sequential steps in the calculation:
1. Multiply by 1000 to convert to μg
2. Divide μg/d by body weight (65 kg)
3. Data read from Figure 2.1
4. Paroxetine μg/l multiplied by 0.15 l/kg/d milk intake
5. Absolute infant dose divided by maternal dose (as %)

were multiplied by a milk intake of 0.15 l/kg/d to yield an absolute infant dose in μg/kg/d. Weight adjusted maternal dose (μg/kg/d) was calculated by dividing the dose (in μg) by an average body weight of 65 kg. Relative infant dose was then calculated according to the equation in section 2.3 above (absolute infant dose *100/maternal dose).

Note that relative infant dose varies over a smaller range (1.1-fold) than absolute infant dose (5.5-fold). This occurs because infant milk intake is assumed to be the same (0.15 l/kg/d) across a five-fold range of maternal dose rates and resulting plasma concentrations. Using the maximum milk concentration in the calculation adopts a very conservative stance in estimating infant dose. A more practical approach is to use the average concentration across the dose interval. While relative infant dose is easily understandable, its interpretation assumes that the maternal dose is within the usual recommended range. For unusually high maternal doses, the absolute infant dose should also be considered. The use of the standard milk intake of 0.15 l/kg/d in these calculations is fairly robust for most situations, but may overestimate the real intake in older infants where supplemental feeding is the norm.

The above calculation of relative infant dose strictly only applies for chronic maternal drug use. Where single drug doses are used in a mother, Bennett[6] recommends a modified calculation scheme.

Finally, direct comparison of a calculated infant dose with the usual therapeutic dose in infants is also helpful in gaining a perspective on infant drug exposure via breast milk[6].

References

1. Besunder JB, Reed MD, Blumer JL. Principles of drug biodisposition in the neonate. A critical evaluation of the pharmacokinetic-pharmacodynamic interface (Part II) [Review]. *Clin Pharmacokinet* 1988;14:261–86

2. Begg EJ. Clinical Pharmacology Essentials. *The Principles Behind the Prescribing Process*. Auckland: Adis International, 2000:34

3. Neville MC, Allen JC, Archer PC, *et al*. Studies in human lactation: milk volume and nutrient composition during weaning and lactogenesis. *Am J Clin Nutr* 1991;54:81–92

4. Bennett PN. Drugs and Human Lactation, 2nd edn. Amsterdam: Elsevier, 1996

5. Stowe ZN, Cohen LS, Hostetter A, *et al*. Paroxetine in human breast milk and nursing infants. *Am J Psychiatry* 2000;157:185–9

6. Bennett PN. Use of the monographs. In: Bennett PN, ed. *Drugs and Human Lactation*, 2nd edn. Amsterdam: Elsevier, 1996:70–4

Chapter 3

Individual risk–benefit analysis

The breastfed infant has nothing to gain from exposure to drugs via his mother's milk and is but an 'innocent bystander'[1]. Thus, the decision to breastfeed should always be an individual risk–benefit analysis, carried out by the mother in collaboration with her medical advisor. The notional safety limit of 10% should be considered carefully in each case and lowered where appropriate.

3.1 Drug safety and breastfeeding

As pointed out above, safety is relative and needs to be individualized. Factors that are worth considering in the context of assessing safety are:

- Infant age – premature and newborn infants are at greater risk;
- Previous long-term experience with the drug in infants – risks may be more confidently predicted when dealing with older drugs that have been used widely;
- Duration of maternal therapy – cessation of breastfeeding may be an option with short-term drug use;

- Presence of active metabolites, which may contribute to either pharmacological or adverse effects in the infant, e.g. fluoxetine in very young infants;
- Drugs that alter milk production; and
- Toxicities that are not dose-related, e.g. allergic sensitization to drugs in milk.

Figure 3.1 presents a schema for the performance of risk–benefit analyses.

3.2 Minimizing the risk

3.2.1 Avoid feeding at C_{max}

It has been suggested that avoiding feeding at times of peak drug concentration in the milk, and feeding only towards the end of the dose interval, may reduce infant exposure. This strategy is really only useful for drugs with very short half-lives that are administered as non-extended-release formulations[2]. In addition, while it may be quite useful for mothers who breastfeed less frequently, in the early postnatal period where feeding is frequent (2–4 hourly) its practicality is questionable.

3.2.2 Avoid drug or delay therapy

Non-essential therapy should be avoided, while elective drug use might reasonably be delayed. Herbal medications with unknown ingredients, and with minimal medical necessity, should be avoided.

3.2.3 Withhold breastfeeding temporarily

This is an excellent strategy where the drug used is moderately hazardous, or where drug use is 'once

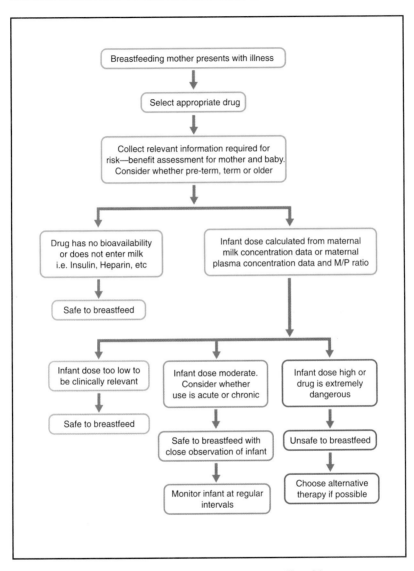

Figure 3.1

Algorithm for the risk–benefit assessment of drug therapy in breastfeeding women

only' or intermittent and the drug half-life is short. Milk produced during the withholding period should be pumped and discarded. This strategy is particularly useful for radioactive or chemotherapeutic medications.

3.2.4 Choose a drug that has low milk concentrations and low relative infant dose
For example, of the newer antidepressants one would choose sertraline, paroxetine or fluvoxamine over fluoxetine or venlafaxine (see section 5.8)[3-6].

3.2.5 Use topical therapy where possible
The route of administration may be manipulated to minimize systemic absorption in the mother. The ultimate test of infant exposure is to measure plasma concentrations of the drug and/or its active metabolites, to observe the infant for medication-related side-effects and to institute regular checks of the infant's growth and development.

3.3 Discontinuation of breastfeeding
This should be necessary only in a selected group of drugs that are therapeutically essential but have significant inherent toxicity. Drugs often included in this category are summarized in Table 3.1.

3.4 Investigation of apparent drug-related adverse reactions
The investigation of apparent drug-related adverse reactions in breastfed infants is an important adjunct to the legitimate use of drugs in breastfeeding women. As with any adverse reaction,

Table 3.1 Drugs that are usually contraindicated in lactating women

Drug	Nature of possible infant risk
Amiodarone	Relative infant dose 4–6% of maternal dose; may accumulate because of very long half-life; adverse cardiovascular and thyroid effects possible[8–9]
Antineoplastic agents	Contraindicated in view of adult adverse effects such as bone marrow suppression, damage to intestinal epithelial cells etc.
Chloramphenicol	Relative infant dose 2% of maternal dose. Blood dyscrasias, aplastic anemia etc. possible but not reported as a result of breastfeeding[10,11]
Ergotamine	Symptoms of ergotism (vomiting and diarrhea) reported[12,13]; potential to inhibit prolactin secretion and hence lower milk production
Gold salts	Relative infant dose varies from 1 to 7%. Relatively long half-lives in adults suggests potential for accumulation. Possiblity of diarrhea, dermatitis, nephrotoxicity and blood dyscrasias[14–16]
Immunosuppressants	Potential for a range of symptoms associated with suppression of the immune system. Cyclosporine appears to be low risk[17–19], but caution is advisable
Lithium	Not recommended as relative infant dose may be up to 56% of maternal dose[20,21]
Phenindione	Relative infant dose calculated at around 18% of maternal dose and abnormal blood coagulation in an infant has been reported[22,23]
Radiopharmaceuticals	The potential for radiation exposure exists and each agent and use circumstance should be carefully considered. See Section 5.9
Retinoids	Secretion into milk is unknown, but is likely to be significant as these drugs are usually very lipid soluble (e.g. isotretinoin). Contraindicated because of the wide range of adverse effects in adults and mutagenic and carcinogenic actions in animals
Tetracyclines (chronic)	While the acute use of tetracyclines for up to 3 weeks is acceptable, chronic use over many months may lead to staining of immature teeth, or changes in epiphyseal bone growth

a detailed investigation of each case is necessary, with due attention being given to alternative diagnoses. Recent *in utero* exposure to drugs should also be considered in premature or very young neonates (e.g. methadone and fluoxetine). Both milk and plasma samples should be obtained from the mother and plasma from the infant so that appropriate laboratory measurements of drug content can be made to assist in the final diagnosis. The final definitive proof is to rechallenge the infant by restarting the maternal drug therapy, but this may well be a difficult decision to make.

References

1. Begg EJ. *Clinical Pharmacology Essentials. The Principles Behind the Prescribing Process.* Auckland: Adis International, 2000:34

2. Wojnar-Horton RE, Hackett LP, Yapp P, *et al.* Distribution and excretion of sumatriptan in human milk. *Br J Clin Pharmacol* 1996;41:217–21

3. Wisner KL, Perel JM, Blumer J. Serum sertraline and N-desmethylsertraline levels in breast-feeding mother-infant pairs. *Am J Psychiatry* 1998;155:690–2

4. Kristensen JH, Ilett KF, Dusci LJ, *et al.* Distribution and excretion of sertraline and N-desmethylsertraline in human milk. *Br J Clin Pharmacol* 1998;45:453–7

5. Kristensen JH, Ilett KF, Hackett LP, *et al.* Distribution and excretion of fluoxetine and norfluoxetine in human milk. *Br J Clin Pharmacol* 1999;48:521–7

6. Kristenson JH, Hackett LP, Kohan R, *et al.* The amount of fluvoxamine in milk is unlikely to be a cause of adverse effects in breastfed infants. *J Hum Lactation* 2001;in press

7. Ilett KF, Hackett LP, Dusci LJ, *et al.* Distribution and excretion of venlafaxine and O-desmethylvenlafaxine in human milk. *Br J Clin Pharmacol* 1998;45:459–62

8. Plomp TA, Vulsma T, de Vijlder JJ. Use of amiodarone during pregnancy. *Eur J Obstet Gynecol Reprod Biol* 1992;43:201–7

9. McKenna WJ, Harris L, Rowland E, *et al.* Amiodarone therapy during pregnancy. *Am J Cardiol* 1983;51:1231–3

10. Havelka J, Hejzlar M, Popov V, *et al.* Excretion of chloramphenicol in human milk. *Chemotherapy* 1968;13:204–11

11. Smadel JE, Woodward TE. Chloramphenicol in the treatment of Tsutsugamushi disease. *J Clin Invest* 1949;1196–215

12. White GJ, White MK. Breastfeeding and drugs in human milk. *Vet Hum Toxicol* 1980;18–24

13. Fomina PI. Untersuchungen uber den Ubergang des aktiven agens des chungen uber den Ubergang des aktiven agens des Muttrkorns in die milch. *Arch Biochem Biophys* 1934;275–7

14. Blau SP. Letter: Metabolism of gold during lactation. *Arth Rheum* 1973;16:777–8

15. Bell RA, Dale IM. Gold secretion in maternal milk. *Arth Rheum* 1976;19:1374

16. Ostensen M, Skavdal K, Myklebust G, et al. Excretion of gold into human breast milk. *Eur J Clin Pharmacol* 1986;31:251–2

17. Flechner SM, Katz AR, Rogers AJ, *et al.* The presence of cyclosporine in body tissues and fluids during pregnancy. *Am J Kidney Dis* 1985;5:60–3

18. Nyberg G, Haljamae U, Frisenette-Fich C, *et al.* Breast-feeding during treatment with cyclosporine. *Transplantation* 1998;65:253–5

19. Ziegenhagen DJ, Crombach G, Dieckmann M, et al. Pregnancy during cyclosporin medication following a kidney transplant. *Deut Med Wochenschr* 1988;113:260–3

20. Llewellyn A, Stowe ZN, Strader JRJ. The use of lithium and management of women with bipolar disorder during pregnancy and lactation [Review]. *J Clin Psychiat* 1998;59 (suppl 6):57–64; discussion 65:57–64

21. Schou M, Amdisen A. Lithium and pregnancy. 3. Lithium ingestion by children breast-fed by women on lithium treatment. *Br Med J* 1973;2:138

22. Goguel M, Noel G, Gilett J-Y, *et al.* Therapeutique anticoagulante laitement. *Rev Fr Gynecol Obstet* 1970;409–12

23. Eckstein HB, Jack B. Breast-feeding and anticoagulant therapy. *Lancet* 1970;i:671–3

Chapter 4

Medication effects
on milk production

4.1 Drugs that inhibit lactation

Apart from the effects of medications on breastfeeding infants, numerous medications also affect the production of breast milk (Table 4.1)[1]. Medications that alter the production of prolactin may profoundly affect milk production, particularly early postpartum. These agents are primarily dopamine agonists and belong to the ergot alkaloid family. Bromocriptine has been used in the past to reduce engorgement and inhibit milk production, although it has been associated with numerous cases of cardiac dysrhythmias, stroke, intracranial bleeding, cerebral edema, convulsions, myocardial infarction and puerperal psychosis[2-6]. A newer analog, cabergoline, has proven much safer and is now recommended for both hyperprolactinemia and inhibition of lactation[7-10]. Doses of 1 mg administered in the early postpartum period will completely inhibit lactation. For established lactation, 0.25 mg twice daily for 2 days has been found to completely inhibit lactation with minimal side-effects[9,10].

Oral contraceptives, particularly those containing estrogens, can suppress lactation significantly if used too early[11-13]. Early postpartum, the use of estrogen-containing oral contraceptives should be avoided and, even when used much later, patients should be advised to observe for changes in milk production. When necessary, progestogen-only oral contraceptives can be used in the first few weeks postpartum. Injectable medroxyprogesterone should be used only after 6 weeks postpartum. Mothers should be placed on oral progestin-only products prior to injecting medroxyprogesterone to determine the effect of progestogens on milk production[13-18].

Table 4.1 Drugs associated with reduced milk production

Estrogens
Bromocriptine
Ergotamine
Cabergoline
Ethanol

4.2 Drugs that stimulate lactation

Dopamine antagonists such as metoclopramide, sulpiride, phenothiazine neuroleptics, risperidone and domperidone are well known to stimulate the production of breast milk. Of these agents, metoclopramide and domperidone may be useful in women with low milk production, and in adoptive mothers who wish to establish lactation.

The most commonly used breast milk stimulant is the gastrokinetic drug metoclopramide. When used early postpartum, it has been found to produce major increases in milk production, particularly in those women with reduced prolactin concentrations[19-22]. Patients should be maintained on metoclopramide until milk production stabilizes and then a slow withdrawal should be instituted. Rapid withdrawal may result in a corresponding reduction in milk production. To date, no untoward effects on the infant have been published. The amount of the metoclopramide in milk varies from 6 to 24 μg/kg/day, a dose significantly less than the maximum clinical dose used in infants for gastroesophageal reflux (0.8 mg/kg/d)[23]. Although not documented in the literature, it is clinically observed that prolonged use of metoclopramide in breastfeeding mothers may lead to profound postpartum depression that rapidly regresses with discontinuation of the drug.

Domperidone, another dopamine antagonist, is perhaps a superior product. Studies show significant elevation of prolactin levels in hypoprolactinemic patients and increased concentrations of milk production in breastfeeding mothers[24-26]. Data from a recent publication by da Silva and colleagues[27] where mothers of premature newborns took domperidone (10 mg three times daily) over a 7-day period are summarized in Table 4.2. Comparing the baseline control day with the other 6 days, mean milk volume increased significantly by 44.5% in the domperidone group compared with a 16.6% increase in the controls. However, inspection of the raw milk volume data in their paper reveals extremely wide inter-patient variability in the response to domperidone. A significant increase in prolactin levels in the treated patients appeared to explain the mechanism for the increased milk volume. The M/P for domperidone was 0.18 and the calculated relative infant dose was 0.04% of the maternal dose. The fact that domperidone does not cross the blood–brain barrier is beneficial as it apparently does not induce neuroleptic side-effects such as extrapyramidal symptoms, sedation and depression[26].

Table 4.2 Effects of domperidone on milk volume and prolactin levels (mean ± standard deviation) in mothers of premature newborns

| Parameter | Placebo | | Domperidone 10 mg thrice daily | |
	Baseline	Study days[a]	Baseline	Study days
Milk volume (ml)	48 ± 63	56 ± 48	113 ± 129	163 ± 128[b]
Prolactin (μg/l)	16 ± 17	18 ± 15	13 ± 8	119 ± 97[c]

[a], days 2–6 for milk volume and day 5 for prolactin; [b], $P < 0.05$ for increase between baseline and study days for placebo (56 ± 48 ml) vs domperidone (8 ± 40 ml); [c], $P = 008$ compared to placebo; data from da Silva et al[27]

References

1. Neville MC, Walsh CT, Bennett PN. Effects of drugs on milk secretion and composition. In: Bennett PN, ed. *Drugs and Human Lactation*, 2nd ed. Amsterdam: Elsevier, 1996:15–46

2. Iffy L, O'Donnell J, Correia J, et al. Severe cardiac dysrhythmia in patients using bromocriptine postpartum. *Am J Ther* 1998;5:111–15

3. Pop C, Metz D, Matei M, et al. Postpartum myocardial infarction induced by Parlodel [in French]. *Arch Mal Coeur Vaiss* 1998;91:1171–4

4. Dutt S, Wong F, Spurway JH. Fatal myocardial infarction associated with bromocriptine for postpartum lactation suppression. *Aust NZ J Obstet Gynaecol* 1998; 38:116–17

5. Webster J. A comparative review of the tolerability profiles of dopamine agonists in the treatment of hyperprolactinaemia and inhibition of lactation. *Drug Saf* 1996;14:228–38

6. O'Shea E. Safety of medications in lactation cessation [Letter]. *Can Fam Physician* 1996;42:616

7. Ferrari C, Piscitelli G, Crosignani PG. Cabergoline: a new drug for the treatment of hyperprolactinaemia. *Hum Reprod* 1995;10: 1647–52

8. Webster J, Piscitelli G, Polli A, et al. The efficacy and tolerability of long-term cabergoline therapy in hyperprolactinaemic disorders: an open, uncontrolled, multicentre study. European Multicentre Cabergoline Study Group. *Clin Endocrinol (Oxf)* 1993;39:323–9

9. European Multicentre Study Group for Cabergoline in Lactation Inhibition. Single dose cabergoline versus bromocriptine in inhibition of puerperal lactation: randomised, double blind, multicentre study. *Br Med J* 1991;302:1367–71

10. Caballero-Gordo A, Lopez-Nazareno N, Calderay M, et al. Oral cabergoline. Single-dose inhibition of puerperal lactation . *J Reprod Med* 1991;36:717–21

11. Booker DE, Pahl IR, Forbes DA. Control of postpartum breast engorgement with oral contraceptives. II. *Am J Obstet Gynecol* 1970;108:240–2

12. Gambrell RDJ. Immediate postpartum oral contraception. *Obstet Gynecol* 1970;36:101–6

13. Booker DE, Pahl IR. Control of postpartum breast engorgement with oral contraceptives. *Am J Obstet Gynecol* 1967;98:1099–101

14. Treffers PE. Breastfeeding and contraception. *Ned Tijdschr Geneeskd* 1999;143: 1900–4

15. Sweezy SR. Contraception for the postpartum woman. *NAACOGS Clin Issu Perinat Womens Health Nurs* 1992;3:209–26

16. Coy JF, Mair CH, Ratkowsky DA. Breastfeeding and oral contraceptives: Tasmanian survey. *Aust Paediatr J* 1983;19:168–71

17. Kelsey JJ. Hormonal contraception and lactation. *J Hum Lact* 1996;12:315–18

18. Visness CM, Rivera R. Progestin-only pill use and pill switching during breastfeeding [Editorial]. *Contraception* 1995;51:279–81

19. Kauppila A, Arvela P, Koivisto M, et al. Metoclopramide and breast feeding: transfer into milk and the newborn. *Eur J Clin Pharmacol* 1983;25:819–23

20. Kauppila A, Kivinen S, Ylikorkala O. A dose response relation between improved lactation and metoclopramide. *Lancet* 1981;1:1175–7

21. Budd SC, Erdman SH, Long DM, et al. Improved lactation with metoclopramide. A case report. *Clin Pediatr (Phila)* 1993;32:53–7

22. Ehrenkranz RA, Ackerman BA. Metoclopramide effect on faltering milk production by mothers of premature infants. *Pediatrics* 1986;78:614–20

23. The Harriet Lane Service Children's Medical and Surgical Center of the Johns Hopkins Hospital. In: Siberry GK, Iannone R, eds. *The Harriet Lane Handbook: A Manual for Pediatric House Officers*, 15th edn. St Louis: Mosby, 2000:771

24. Petraglia F, De L, V, Sardelli S, et al. Domperidone in defective and insufficient lactation. *Eur J Obstet Gynecol Reprod Biol* 1985;19:281–7

25. Hofmeyr GJ, Van Iddekinge B, Blott JA. Domperidone: secretion in breast milk and effect on puerperal prolactin levels. *Br J Obstet Gynaecol* 1985;92:141–4

26. Hofmeyr GJ, Van Iddekinge B. Domperidone and lactation [Letter]. *Lancet* 1983;1:647

27. da Silva OP, Knoppert DC, Angelini MM, Forret PA. Effect of domperidone on milk production in mothers of premature newborns: a randomized, double-blind, placebo-controlled trial. *CMAJ* 2001;164:17–21

Chapter 5

Commentary on selected drug classes

5.1 Analgesics

Analgesics are the most commonly used medication in breastfeeding mothers and data for selected drugs are shown in Table 5.1.

5.1.1 Nonspecific anti-inflammatory drugs

While not all of the nonspecific anti-inflammatory drugs (NSAIDs) have been studied in breastfeeding mothers, the transfer of most NSAIDs into human milk is minimal. Ibuprofen is considered an ideal analgesic, because of its short half-life and its very low milk concentrations (generally less than 0.5 mg/l)[1]. Ketorolac, another popular but controversial analgesic is poorly transferred to milk, with concentrations varying from 5 to 7.3 μg/l of milk[3]. The estimated dose to an infant following oral administration to a mother would be approximately 1.2 μg/kg/d, a dose that is unlikely to affect even a newborn infant[3].

Longer half-life NSAIDs, such as naproxen, produce low milk concentrations and have a low potential for toxicity; if used chronically they may lead to gastric

Table 5.1 Maternal, infant doses and relative infant dose for selected analgesic agents

Drug	Maternal dose	Infant dose (μg/kg/d)	Relative infant dose (%)	Clinical significance[a]	References
Nonsteroidal anti-inflammatory drugs					
Ibuprofen	1600 mg/d	150[b]	0.6	None detected in infants; no adverse effects; safe	1,2
Ketorolac	40 mg/d	1.2[b]	0.16–0.4	Dose too low to effect infant; no adverse effects; safe	3
Naproxen	750 mg/d	355[b]	3.0	Long half-life; may accumulate in infant. Bleeding, diarrhea reported in one infant. Short-term use acceptable; avoid chronic use	4
Indomethacin	75–300 mg/d	17[b]	0.4	Low levels in milk; plasma levels low to undetectable in infants; probably safe but caution with chronic administration	5
Opioids					
Morphine	90 mg/d	75[b]	5.8	Oral bioavailability poor; milk levels generally low; considered safe; observe for sedation	6,7
Methadone	20–180 mg/d	17[b], 36[b], 22[b], 14[b]	2.6, 5.6, 2.4, 1.0	Neonatal abstinance syndrome occurs in many infants in the first 2 weeks of life. Breastfeeding is safe but does not always deliver enough drug to prevent withdrawal	8–10
Pethidine (meperidine)	50 mg/4–6 h	41[b]	1	Neurobehavioral delay, sedation noted from long half-life metabolite; avoid	6,11,12
Fentanyl	2 μg/kg iv	0.06[b]	< 3	Milk levels low; no untoward effects from exposure to milk	13,14

[a] , safe – term is relative and infants must always be observed closely; [b] , calculated from C_{max}

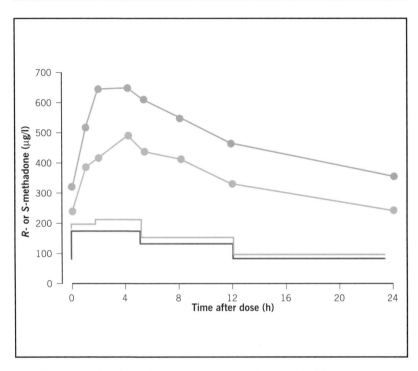

and hemorrhagic side-effects in the breastfed infant[15]. Using naproxen for a few days would not be contraindicated, but prolonged use is questionable. Indomethacin was associated with seizures in one infant[16] although another study in 16 infants showed minimal transfer (relative infant dose = 0.11–0.18%) and no adverse effects[5].

5.1.2 Methadone

Methadone is used widely in the treatment of opiate addiction and often encountered in both pregnancy and lactation. The M/P for racemic methadone ranges from 0.24 to 0.83[8,9,17,18] and mean relative infant dose varies from 1.0 to 5.6% of the maternal

Figure 5.1
Concentrations of methadone enantiomers in milk (R- ●; S- ●) and plasma (R- ●; S- ●) for a methadone maintenance client with mature milk production – daily dose of 75 mg racemic methadone. M/PAUC for R-methadone = 0.39 and S-methadone = 0.24. Data from with permission from Blackwell Science Publishers, Oxford, UK from Begg EJ, Malpas TJ, Hackett LP, et al. Distribution of R- and S-methadone into human milk at steady state during ingestion of medium to high doses. Br J Clin Pharmacol 2001;in press

dose[8,9,19]. Begg and colleagues[9] have investigated the transfer of the *R*- and *S*-enantiomers of methadone into human milk and data from one patient in their series are shown in Figure 5.1. *R*-methadone has approximately 50 times the potency of *S*-methadone as an agonist at the μ-opioid receptor[20] and is also a more potent blocker of the reuptake of serotonin in the brain[21]. By contrast, *S*-methadone has non-competitive antagonist activity at the *N*-methyl-D-aspartate (NMDA) receptor[22], which is excitatory for functions such as respiration[23]. The M/P for *R*-methadone (0.64 ± 0.17; mean ± 95% CI) was significantly higher than that for *S*-methadone (0.36 ± 0.1), an observation that may be due to the lower plasma protein binding of the *R*-enantiomer[24]. Relative infant dose was 3.27 ± 1.22% (mean ± 95% CI) for *R*-methadone and 2.05 ± 0.59% for *S*-methadone.

Neonatal abstinence syndrome (NAS) occurs in 60–90% of newborns whose mothers take methadone throughout pregnancy[25–27]. In most cases, the methadone received in breast milk is insufficient to prevent the NAS[28] and treatment of the infant with other drugs, such as morphine or phenobarbitone, may be necessary in the early postnatal period. In a recent study by McCarthy and Posey, patients receiving methadone doses of 25–180 mg/d produced milk methadone concentrations ranging from 27 to 260 μg/l with a mean for the group of 95 μg/l[19]. Assuming a daily milk intake of 475 ml, the average infant daily methadone oral dose can be calculated to be approximately 0.05 mg/day. This corresponds to an average relative infant dose of 0.97%, and readily illustrates why NAS occurs frequently. Nevertheless, individual cases may be different and, in another study in one infant, an abrupt cessation of breastfeeding was associated with an acute withdrawal[29]. Apart from problems with NAS from *in utero* exposure, methadone use during breastfeeding has not been associated with adverse outcomes except for one case where there was a possible association between maternal methadone use and the death of a breastfed infant[30]. However, in this case, the plasma concentration in the infant was 400 μg/l, which is in the adult therapeutic range and strongly suggestive of exogenous administration of methadone to the infant.

5.1.3 Morphine

The amount of morphine that transfers into milk has long been controversial, but is believed to be subclinical. Older studies using poorer methodologies found that the amount in milk was low or undetectable[31,32]. In another study, the highest morphine concentration in breast milk following two epidural doses (4 mg each) was only 82 μg/l at 30 min after dose[6]. The highest breast milk concentration following 15 mg intravenously or intramuscularly was only 500 μg/l. Other data from Robieux and colleagues[33] suggest that the concentrations transferred to the infant ranged from 10 to 100 μg/l. In another more recent study of women who received morphine or pethidine via patient-controlled analgesia pumps for 12–48 h postpartum, the concentration of morphine in breast milk ranged from 50 to 60 µg/l and did not affect the infants[6]. Overall, combined with its low oral bioavailability (< 25%) and minimal milk levels, most studies suggest that morphine is not a significant hazard to breastfeeding infants so long as the maternal doses are low to moderate, and the infant is reasonably stable.

5.1.4 Pethidine

Small amounts of pethidine penetrate into breast milk. Concentrations in milk vary from 0.13 mg/l[11] to 0.275 mg/l[12]. Although the concentrations of pethidine transferred via milk appear low, neurobehavioral depression has been reported[6].

5.1.5 Fentanyl

The transfer of fentanyl into human milk is low. In women receiving a total dose of 50–400 µg fentanyl intravenously during labor, the concentration of fentanyl in milk was exceedingly low, generally below the limit of detection (< 0.05 µg/l)[13]. Under most clinical conditions, the transfer of fentanyl into milk and subsequently to the infant is minimal.

5.2 Anticonvulsants

Most of the older anticonvulsants have been studied in breastfeeding mothers and in general do not pose a problem for a breastfed infant. Selected drugs of this group are reviewed below and in Table 5.2.

5.2.1 Magnesium sulfate

Magnesium transfer to the fetus *in utero* is well known and has led to significant sedation in

Table 5.2 Maternal, infant doses and relative infant dose for selected anticonvulsant agents

Drug	Maternal dose	Infant dose (μg/kg/d)	Relative infant dose (%)	Clinical significance[a]	References
Carbamazepine	800 mg/d 1000 mg/d	270[b] 345[b]	2.3 2.4	Most studies show no effect of medication on breastfed infants. Safe, but observe for sedation	34,35
Lamotrigine	200 mg/d 300 mg/d	522[b] 976[b]	18.2 22.7	Dose is very high; limited studies show no untoward effects on infants. Avoid if possible. Observe infant closely if used	36–38
Magnesium sulfate	4 g stat; 1 g/h (day one)	1845[d]	0.5	Magnesium transfer to milk is minimal; oral bioavailability is < 15%; day 2, milk levels of Mg^{++} in treated and untreated groups identical	39
Phenobarbitone	120 mg/d	411[b]	24	Milk concentrations may be significant; use caution; observe for sedation; but may continue to breastfeed with close observation	40
Phenytoin	400 mg/d	442	7.7	Studies are conflicting; average milk levels are low; no untoward effects reported in infants; safe	41
Valproic acid	300–2400 mg/d 2170 mg/d	285[c] 810[b]	1.6 2.6	Milk concentrations are low compared to maternal dose; no untoward effects noted; safe with close monitoring	42,43

[a], safe – term is relative & infants must always be observed closely; [b], calculated from c_{max}; [c], calculated from average of c_{max}; [d], calculated from difference between treated and untreated milk magnesium levels

newborns. Subsequent observations have suggested that the use of magnesium sulfate may be related to poorer milk production and a later onset of lactation, but this has not been proven. However, the transfer of magnesium sulfate into human milk is minimal, even following substantial intravenous doses[39]. Because the oral bioavailability of magnesium is only 15% or less, the actual dose absorbed by the infant is likely to be very small. The use of intravenous magnesium sulfate postnatally is not a contraindication to breastfeeding.

5.2.2 Phenobarbitone

Fortunately, phenobarbitone is poorly absorbed in the neonate. In addition, its protein binding is lower than in adults, and thus its volume of distribution is likely to be higher, with the end result of lower concentrations in the brain. With milk concentrations averaging about 3 mg/l following a dose of 120 mg daily, phenobarbitone does not seem to accumulate in full-term or older breastfed infants[40]. However, phenobarbitone may have contributed to one case of suffocation, and close observation is recommended[44]. It is advisable to monitor phenobarbitone plasma concentrations in both the mother and her breastfed infant during therapy, and to monitor infant weight gain and behavior early after the initiation of therapy.

5.2.3 Phenytoin

The transfer of phenytoin into human milk is negligible. The effect on the infant is generally considered minimal if the maternal plasma concentrations are kept at the low end of the usual therapeutic range (10 mg/l). Milk concentrations in the range of 0.8 to 6 mg/l have been reported[45].

5.2.4 *Valproic acid*

Valproic acid transfers into human milk at very low concentrations, generally less than 3% of the maternal dose. Average concentrations in breast milk range from 0.17 to 0.47 mg/l of milk[40,46]. To date, no untoward effects have been reported.

5.2.5 *Gabapentin*

No data are available for this newer anticonvulsant. However, owing to its limited toxicity and minimal sedative properties in adults, it has been used in a small number of breastfeeding patients and no untoward effects have been reported (TW Hale, unpublished communications).

5.2.6 *Lamotrigine*

At present only two patients have been studied and with milk concentrations varying from 3.5 mg/l[37] to 6.5 mg/l[38], the relative infant dose was 18–23%. Both authors suggest caution in the use of lamotrigine during breastfeeding. An additional reason for avoiding lamotrigine is that severe rash and Stevens–Johnson syndrome have been reported following its administration to older children[47].

5.3 Antihistamines

Studies reporting the transfer of antihistamines into human milk are limited. While many of the older antihistamines induce significant sedation in adults and children, they have not been reported to sedate breastfed infants. However, it is advisable to use the new non-sedating antihistamines where possible. Current data for loratadine suggest milk concentrations are quite low and the infant dose of loratadine, and its active metabolite, would be only 0.46% of the administered maternal dose[48]. Fexofenadine, the active metabolite of terfenadine is another good choice. After usual therapeutic doses of the parent terfenadine, the maximum concentration of fexofenadine observed was 60 μg/l[49], with a relative infant dose of 0.45%. No data are available on cetirizine, but it is probably another good choice because of its limited sedative properties, and the fact that it is widely used in older infants.

5.4 Antibiotics and antivirals

Selected drugs of this group are reviewed below and in Table 5.3.

5.4.1 Penicillins and cephalosporins

Virtually all of the penicillins and cephalosporins have been studied and have been found to produce only trace concentrations in milk[51,54,57,79-81]. The only likely consequences of these amounts in milk are a change in the gastrointestinal flora, or allergic sensitization, although these rarely occur. Infants should be observed for symptoms that might suggest overgrowth with *Clostridium difficile* or *Candida albicans*.

5.4.2 Aminoglycosides

The aminoglycosides are quite polar molecules, have very low oral bioavailability and do not pass into milk in significant quantities. Following a total intramuscular dose of gentamicin (240 mg/day), milk concentrations were generally less than 0.5 mg/l of milk[58]. Plasma concentrations were below the limit of detection in half of the infants. Because of its low oral bioavailability, the absorption of gentamicin in the breastfed infant is likely to be minimal. Again, changes in gastrointestinal flora are possible, but unlikely.

5.4.3 Tetracyclines

The concentration of most tetracyclines in milk is low, and ranges from 1.2 to 2.6 mg/l[82]. While the bioavailability of the older tetracyclines, when dissolved in milk, is quite low owing to chelation with calcium, the newer tetracyclines, such as doxycycline and minocycline, are the least bound to calcium (only 20%), and their bioavailability in adults is only slowed and not significantly decreased. Therefore the bioavailability of doxycycline in breastfeeding infants could be significant. Thus, some have suggested that tetracyclines may be used for short periods (e.g. 2–3 weeks) without significant risk of staining the teeth. However, long-term use, such as for acne, is not advisable during breastfeeding.

5.4.4 Antifungals

The azole antifungals (e.g. fluconazole, ketoconazole, miconazole) have seen greater use in some communities mainly because of the development of resistance to nystatin. In some breastfeeding mothers *C. albicans* has been found

Table 5.3 Maternal, infant doses and relative infant dose for selected antimicrobial agents

Drug	Maternal dose	Infant dose (μg/kg/d)	Relative infant dose (%)	Clinical significance[a]	References
Penicillins					
Ampicillin	4 g/d	137[c]	0.24	Safe; observe for changes in intestinal flora	50
Amoxicillin	1 g/d	195[b]	1.3	Safe; observe for changes in intestinal flora	51
Cloxacillin	500 mg	60[b]	0.8	Safe; observe for changes in intestinal flora	52
Dicloxacillin	250 mg	45[b]	1.2	Safe; observe for changes in intestinal flora	53
Cephalosporins					
Cefazolin	2 g/d	226[b]	0.8	Safe; observe for changes in intestinal flora	54
Cefoperazone	1 g/d	135[b]	0.9	Safe; observe for changes in intestinal flora Personal communication, Pfizer-Roerig Laboratories, 1996	
Cefotaxime	1 g/d	48[b]	0.3	Safe; observe for changes in intestinal flora	55
Cefoxitin	2–4 g/d	135[b]	0.2	Safe; observe for changes in intestinal flora	56
Ceftazidime	6 g/d	780[b]	0.9	Safe; observe for changes in intestinal flora	57
Ceftriaxone	1 g/d	132[c]	0.9	Safe; observe for changes in intestinal flora	51
Cephalexin	1 g/d	75[b]	0.5	Safe; observe for changes in intestinal flora	51
Aminoglycosides					
Gentamicin	240 mg	73.5[b]	2.1	Safe; observe for changes in intestinal flora	58
Streptomycin	1 g/d	90[b]	0.6	Safe; observe for changes in intestinal flora	59
Macrolides					
Erythromycin	1.2 g/d	240[b]	1.4	Safe; observe for changes in intestinal flora; hypertonic pyloric stenosis reported in one case Personal communication, Pfizer-Roerig Laboratories, 1996	60
Azithromycin	1g stat + 500mg/d	420[b]	5.8	Safe; observe for change in intestinal flora	61

continued over

Figure 5.3 continued

	Dose		Ratio	Comment	Ref
Quinolones					
Ciprofloxacin	1.5 g/d	568[b]	2.6	Probably safe, but one case of pseudomembranous colitis reported; observe for changes in gut flora	62–64
	0.5 g/d	147[b]	2.0		
Ofloxacin	0.8 g/d	361[b]	3.2	Probably safe, but observe for changes in intestinal flora	62
Miscellaneous					
Acyclovir	1 g/d	159[b]	1.1	Infant dose low; safe	65,66
	4 g/d	872[b]	1.5		
Clindamycin	2.4 g/d	570[b]	1.6	Probably safe, but observe for changes in intestinal flora. Pseudomembranous colitis reported in one infant	67,68
Doxycycline	0.2 g/d	115[d]	4	Infant dose low; bioavailability poor; safe for acute use; do not use chronically	69
Fluconazole	150 mg	440[b]	17.6	No untoward effects have been reported. However, infant dose is high and caution is suggested in very young neonates	70
Isoniazid	0.7 g/d	1350[b]	13.5	Caution; monitoring of infant for liver toxicity and neuritis recommended	59
Metronidazole	1.2 g/d	2325[b]	13	No major untoward effects have been reported; dose via milk significantly less than pediatric therapeutic dose (15mg/kg/d). With high doses, discontinue breastfeeding for 12–24 hours after dose	71–73
	0.6 g/d	855[b]	9.9		
	1.2 g/d	2160[b]	12.6		
	2 g/d Stat	8550[b]	29		
Nitrofurantoin	400 mg	None detected		Safe; no untoward effects reported; caution for infants with G6PD	74,75
	0.8 g/d	75[b]	0.7		
Rifampicin	0.45 g/d	735[b]	11	Probably safe; minimal data available	76
Tetracycline	2 g/d	387[b]	1.35	Short-term use safe; bioavailability in milk is low to nil; caution with long-term use	77
Vancomycin	2 g/d	1905[b]	6.6	Safe; oral bioavailability low to nil. Observe for changes in intestinal flora	78

[a], safe: term is relative and infants must always be observed closely; [b], calculated from C_{max}; [c], calculated from average of C_{max}; [d], calculated from average concentration over dose interval

in milk and on damaged nipples[83-85], making breastfeeding extremely painful. While topical therapy with nystatin, clotrimazole or miconazole may work in some cases, systemic therapy with fluconazole may be required for more severe infections of the breast. Although there is significant controversy about the presence of *C. albicans* in breast tissues[86], some patients respond poorly to topical therapy and much better to systemic therapy with fluconazole or ketoconazole. Doses of 100–200 mg/d of fluconazole for 14–21 days may be useful in patients with candida-like symptoms who have not responded to topical therapy. One chronic dosing study reported milk concentrations of up to 2.93 mg/l, which corresponds to a relative infant dose of 17.6%[70]. Even so, the absolute dose transferred to the infant is significantly less than the therapeutic dose used in full-term neonates (3–6 mg/kg/d)[87]. There are no reports of changes in liver function following exposure to these doses in breastfed infants. However, caution should be used, particularly in very young neonates where renal function is not fully developed. For single-dose therapy exposure would correspondingly be lower and withholding breastfeeding for 24–48 h could essentially prevent exposure. Caution also may be appropriate where these drugs are used in an infant receiving therapeutic doses of cisapride because of the theoretical possibility of drug interactions.

5.4.5 Sulfonamides

The sulfonamides can be used in breastfeeding patients, although there is some risk of displacing bilirubin from its albumin binding site and worsening kernicterus in the early postnatal period. Sulfonamides can be used with relative safety in mothers of older breastfed infants. Sulfisoxazole has been studied and milk levels are less than 1% of the maternal dose[88]. Trimethoprim, which is commonly encountered together with sulfamethoxazole in co-trimoxazole preparations, does enter milk but the concentrations are extremely low[89].

5.4.6 Fluoroquinolones

Because they have been implicated in arthropathy, fluoroquinolones generally are contraindicated in pediatric patients. Ciprofloxacin concentrations in human milk vary over a wide range[62,63,90] and have been identified as causing pseudomembranous colitis in one infant[64]. Studies of the newer quinolones suggest that ofloxacin concentrations may be somewhat lower than those of ciprofloxacin[62]. Therefore preferred fluoroquinolones for breastfeeding mothers would include ofloxacin or its congener levofloxacin. While it is very unlikely that the amount of quinolones present in milk could induce arthropathy, changes in gastrointestinal flora are possible.

5.4.7 Erythromycin and macrolides

Erythromycin is transferred into milk, but the concentrations are low. Doses of 2 g daily produce milk concentrations of only 1.6–3.2 mg/l[60]. Azithromycin has also been studied and milk concentrations also are low. The predicted dose to the infant would be approximately 0.4 mg/kg/day[61].

To date there are no data for clarithromycin. Caution may be appropriate where these drugs are used in an infant receiving therapeutic doses of cisapride because of the theoretical possibility of drug interactions.

5.4.8 Metronidazole

Metronidazole is one of the most commonly used antibiotics in neonates and has been extensively studied in breastfeeding mothers. Concentrations in milk are low to moderate depending on the dose and route of administration. Following an oral dose of 400 mg three times daily, peak milk concentrations were 15.5 mg/l[71]. At this dose, infant plasma concentrations varied from 1.2 to 2.4 mg/l, concentrations which are below the usual therapeutic range (5.5–6.7 mg/l)[91]. Milk concentrations following intravenous administration have not been reported, but with a short withholding period of a few hours to avoid the peak, the infant dose should not be much different than that following oral administration. Older suggestions of mutagenicity in rodents have never been documented in humans. Intravaginal use of metronidazole produces only 2% of the mean peak serum concentrations of a 500 mg oral tablet, which would be of no concern in breastfeeding[92]. High single doses such as the 2 g oral dose used for trichomoniasis produce high milk concentrations, but these are not sustained[73]. Milk and plasma concentrations fall rapidly, and after a 12–24 h withholding period infants can safely resume breastfeeding. Few, if any side-effects attributable to metronidazole have been reported, other than a slight metallic taste in the milk, and with the above caveats, it is considered safe to use in breastfeeding mothers.

5.4.9 Acyclovir

Acyclovir concentrations in milk are low, and following doses as high as 4 g/day, breast milk concentrations ranged from 4.2 to 5.8 mg/l, corresponding to an average infant dose of 0.73 mg/kg/d (relative infant dose 1.3%)[66]. This is well below doses commonly used in infants (15–45 mg/kg/d)[93] and is unlikely to cause adverse effects. In addition, infant exposure would be expected to be decreased because of the low oral bioavailability of acyclovir (approximately 15%). Figure 5.2 shows a simulation of plasma and milk acyclovir concentrations at steady-state for an oral dose regimen of 800 mg three times daily. A plasma half-life of 2.6 h and volume of distribution of 0.7 l/kg[94], and a milk half-life of 2.8 h[65] have been used in the simulation. The figure shows that the milk and plasma concentration-time profiles for this drug do not change in parallel, with the plasma peak at around 50 min and the milk peak at around 3 h after dose. Profiles of this kind can result in highly variable estimates for M/P ratio. For example, M/P based on single plasma and milk data pairs at the trough, plasma peak and milk peak times are 12, 0.6 and 4.8 respectively, while M/P based on AUC data is around 3.1.

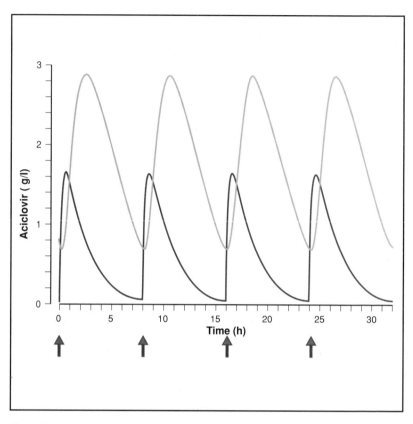

Figure 5.2

Simulated plasma (red line) and milk (green line) concentration-time profiles at steady-state for acyclovir for a 800 mg oral dose given three times daily (at arrows).

5.4.10 Valaciclovir

Valaciclovir is a prodrug of acyclovir. It is rapidly absorbed and has a higher bioavailability than acyclovir (approximately 55%) and maternal plasma concentrations that are 3–5 times higher than with acyclovir[95]. Acyclovir is therefore preferred over valaciclovir for breastfeeding mothers.

5.5 Antihypertensives

Selected drugs for this group are reviewed below and summarized in Table 5.4.

5.5.1 Angiotensin-converting enzyme inhibitors

Angiotensin-converting enzyme (ACE) inhibitors are generally considered to be a risk for neonates. Newborns have poor control of blood pressure and several cases of hypotension and renal failure have been reported from the perinatal use of ACE inhibitors[116]. The milk concentrations of these drugs in breastfeeding mothers have been studied for captopril, enalapril and quinapril, and only minimal concentrations were found in milk[103-105]. In a single dose study by Begg and colleagues[105] where 20 mg of quinapril was administered to volunteer lactating women, plasma quinapril was not quantifiable 6 h after dose (limit of detection 5 μg/l), and quinapril in milk averaged 27.9 mg/l in the first 4 h after dose and was undetectable (limit of detection 5 μg/l) at later times (Figure 5.3). The authors point out that infant exposure was very low and that even this low level could be avoided by breastfeeding 4 h after dose. No adverse events were noted, and these agents are therefore preferred[103]. Nevertheless, infants should be monitored frequently when maternal ACE inhibitor treatment is necessary, particularly in the early postnatal period.

5.5.2 β-adrenoceptor blockers

The transfer of various β-blockers into breast milk has been extensively studied. Because some β-blockers have been associated with cyanosis and bradycardia in breastfed infants[96,117] choosing the most appropriate β-blocker for the breastfeeding mother is important. Interestingly, it is the more lipid soluble β-blockers propranolol[102,118,119] and

Table 5.4 Maternal, infant doses and relative infant dose for selected antihypertensive agents

Drug	Maternal dose	Infant dose (µg/kg/d)	Relative infant dose (%)	Clinical significance[a]	References
Beta blockers					
Acebutolol	1.2 g/d	618[b]	3.6	Hypotension, bradycardia have been reported; use caution	96
	0.6 g/d	81[b]	0.9		
Atenolol	100 mg/d	95[b]	6.6	Bradycardia, cyanosis reported in one case; caution recommended; use with close observation	97–99
	100 mg/d	270[b]	18.9		
		255[b]	17.8		
Labetalol	1200 mg/d	99[b]	0.6	Safe; observe for hypotension, bradycardia	100
Metoprolol	200 mg/d	42[b]	1.5	Safe; observe for hypotension, bradycardia	101
Propranolol	2.61 mg/kg/d	5.3[d]	0.2	Safe; observe for hypotension, bradycardia	102
ACE inhibitors					
Captopril	300 mg/d	0.4[c]	0.01	Caution early postpartum; otherwise safe	103
Enalapril	20 mg/d	0.88	0.31 (0.12)[e]	Caution early postpartum; otherwise safe	104
Quinapril	20mg single dose	4.2[d]	1.5	Caution early postpartum; otherwise safe	105
Calcium channel blockers					
Diltiazem	240 mg	34.5[b]	1	Probably safe; only limited data available; observe for hypotension	106
Nifedipine	10 mg/d	1.54[b]	1	Safe; infant dose very low; no untoward effects reported	107–109
	20 mg/d	6.9[b]	2.4		
	30 mg/d	8.0[b]	1.8		
Verapamil	240 mg/d	3.87[b]	0.1	Safe; observe for hypotension	110,111
	320 mg/d	45[b]	1		
Miscellaneous antihypertensives					
Methyldopa	500 mg/d	99[b]	1.4	Safe; observe for hypotension, gynecomastia	112,113
	1000 mg/d	171[b]	1.1		
Clonidine	391 µg/d	5.58[b]	7.5	Clonidine levels in infant were low to mid range. Caution; observe for hypotension	114,115
	75 µg/d	1.07[b]	8.4		

[a], safe: term is relative and infants must always be observed closely; [b], calculated from Cmax; [c], calculated from average of Cmax; [d], calculated from average concentration over dose interval; [e], includes active metabolite

metoprolol[101] that produce the lowest milk concentrations. The transfer of labetolol to milk also is minimal, with a reported infant dose of only 99 μg/kg/d[100]. The relative infant doses of acebutolol[96] and atenolol[97] are higher with reports of hypotension in breastfed infants.

5.5.3 Hydralazine
Hydralazine has been studied in breastfeeding mothers and the milk concentrations are quite low[120]. The theoretical dose to the infant would be approximately 25 μg/kg/d, a dose that is considerably less than the pediatric therapeutic dose of 1 mg/kg/day[120].

5.5.4 Calcium channel blockers
Nifedipine concentrations in milk are low, and the drug has been used extensively to control blood pressure and other syndromes in breastfeeding mothers[107-109]. Milk concentrations were dependent on dose and timing, but the dose to the infant via milk was generally less than 8 μg/kg/day[109]. Two studies of verapamil use in breastfeeding mothers have reported a relative infant dose of 0.1–1%[110,121].

5.5.5 Methyldopa
Methyldopa concentrations in milk are low[112,113]. Following doses as high as 1000 mg/d, milk concentrations were only 1.1 mg/l. While gynecomastia has been reported in adults, there are no published reports of this adverse effect in breastfed infants. However, we are aware of a single case of a 2-week-old female infant with prominent

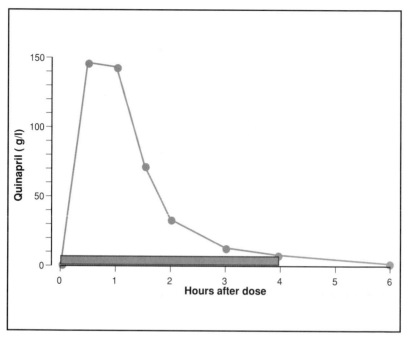

Figure 5.3

Quinapril concentrations in plasma (●) and milk (red shaded area) following a 20 mg single oral dose to a lactating woman. Redrawn with permission from Blackwell Science Publishers, Oxford, UK from Begg EJ, Robson RA, Gardiner SJ, *et al*. Quinapril and its metabolite quinaprilat in human milk. *Br J Clin Pharmacol* 2001:478–81

gynecomastia, who regressed when the mother ceased taking methyldopa (TW Hale, personal communication).

5.6 Steroids and hormones

Corticosteroids transfer poorly into human milk. Following moderately high doses of prednisone (80 mg), the calculated amount the infant would ingest from milk is only 10 μg/kg, which is approximately 10% of the endogenous production level[122]. In one patient receiving 120 mg prednisone daily, breast milk concentrations ranged from 54 to 627 μg/l at 30 min and 2 h respectively after dose[123]. To date, no adverse events have been reported in breastfed infants following maternal treatment with prednisone. However, breastfeeding following chronic high dose prednisone or methylprednisolone should be questioned. Infant exposure to single high doses of methylprednisolone (e.g. 1–2 g intravenously for multiple sclerosis) may be limited by an appropriate withholding period of 1–2 days (Figure 5.4). Since no milk concentrations are available, the figure shows simulated plasma concentrations of methylprednisolone at either 120 mg or 1 g daily as a 20 min infusion. Assuming a conservative M/P value of 0.25, the calculated maximum infant doses at 8, 12 and 24 h after the 1 g administration to the mother were 8.5, 1.2 and 0.002 μg/kg/d respectively. By comparison, anti-inflammatory/immunosuppressive therapeutic doses of methylprednisolone used in infants are an order of magnitude greater at 0.5–1.7 mg/kg/d[125]. Therefore, it is likely that pumping and discarding milk for a period of 8–24 h following a 1 g dose of methylprednisolone would dramatically reduce infant exposure via breast milk. This example shows what can be done when milk concentration data on a particular drug are not available. While such calculations may be helpful for individual cases, the ultimate goal must be to provide quantitative data on methylprednisolone concentrations in milk.

5.7 Thyroid and antithyroid drugs

Levothyroxine is known to transfer poorly into human milk. While the actual amount in milk is controversial, it is invariably quite low[126–128]. Liothyronine concentrations are apparently somewhat higher (0.1 μg/l)[128]. These data indicate

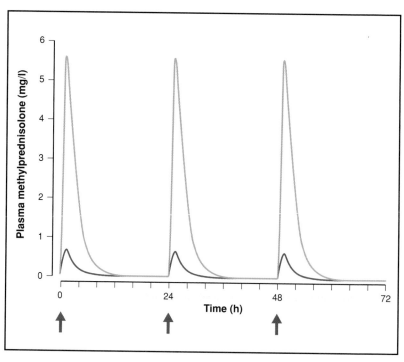

Figure 5.4

Simulated plasma concentrations of methylprednisolone following three consecutive daily intravenous infusion (over 30 min, at arrows) doses of 120 mg (red line) or 1 g (green line) detailing rapid decline and disappearance of drug from the plasma compartment. Mean pharmacokinetic descriptors for the simulation were taken from Vree *et al*[124]. Assuming a conservative estimate of 0.25 for M/P, estimates of relative infant dose can be made at various times after dose, and used as a guide to when breastfeeding may be safely resumed (see Section 5.6)

that transfer of thyroid hormones through the mammary gland is different for T4 and T3. Moreover, since drug transfer is low, human milk alone does not provide sufficient thyroxine for the needs of the hypothyroid breastfed infant[127–129].

In hyperthyroid states, both propylthiouracil (PTU) and methimazole have been studied. PTU concentrations in milk are approximately 10-fold lower than in the maternal plasma and the amount excreted in milk is minimal. Following a dose of 400 mg, the average amount of PTU secreted over 4 h was only 99 μg[129]. One study using radiolabeled PTU showed that only 0.08% of a dose of PTU transferred into milk over 24 h[130]. No changes in infant thyroid function have been reported following maternal use of PTU.

Following administration of carbimazole, concentrations of its active metabolite methimazole in milk are similar to those in plasma[131]. A review of the limited data available for methimazole after administration of carbimazole suggests that the relative infant dose could vary by 2–12% and that breastfeeding is safe provided the carbimazole dose does not exceed 30 mg/d[132]. In addition, no change in infant thyroid function was noted following the maternal use of methimazole or carbimazole in a study of 139 infants and their mothers[133].

5.8 Psychotherapeutic agents

Selected drugs of this group are reviewed below and commonly used drugs are also summarized in Table 5.5.

5.8.1 Sedatives

Diazepam[152,153,157,158], lorazepam[154,155,159], clonazepam[160], nitrazepam[156], midazolam[156] and oxazepam[161] have all been studied in breastfeeding mothers. The amounts transferred into human milk are low, and intermittent single doses do not pose an overt hazard to the breastfed infant. However, when used chronically, diazepam, lorazepam and clonazepam may occasionally accumulate and cause sedation in the breastfed infant. As might be predicted, the longer the half-life of the benzodiazepine, the higher the probability of infant sedation[156]. The intermittent use of diazepam, midazolam or lorazepam has not been associated with significant sedation in breastfed infants and, in

Table 5.5 Maternal, infant doses and relative infant dose for selected psychotherapeutic agents

Drug	Maternal dose	Infant dose (μg/kg/d)	Relative infant dose (%)	Clinical significance[a]	References
Antidepressants					
Citalopram	20–60 mg/d	14.6[d]	3.7 (1.4)[e]	Not detected in infants; no adverse effects; safe	134
Fluoxetine	20–80 mg/d (0.51 mg/kg/d)	19.5[c]	3.4 (3.5)[e]	Fluoxetine & norfluoxetine found in 55–77% of infants; not recommended in pre-term or very young neonates	135,136
	7–65 mg/d (0.17–0.85 mg/kg/d)	44[b]	4.4 (5.6)[e]		
Fluvoxamine	200 mg/d (2.86 mg/kg/d)	14	0.5	No adverse effects in 2 infants; probably safe	137,138
	100 mg/d	26[c]	0.52		
Nefazodone	200 mg/d	20[b]	0.3	Very small number of infants studied. Probably safe but more data needed. Caution with pre-term infants	139,140
	300 mg/d	54[b]	0.3		
Paroxetine	20–30 mg/d	4[d]	1.4	Not detected in infants; no adverse effects; safe	141,142
	10–50 mg/d	2.6–15[b]	1.7–2.3		
Sertraline	50 mg/d	9[d]	0.9 (1.3)[e]	Not detected in infants in one study & low levels in some infants in the other; no adverse effects; safe	143,144
	25–200 mg/d	2.3–15[c]	0.3–1.9[e]		
Venlafaxine	150–450 mg/d (6.1 mg/kg/d)	85[d]	3.5, (4.1)[e]	O-desmethyl metabolite detected in 50% of infants; no adverse effects reported; use cautiously and monitor metabolite in infant serum	145,146
	(225–300 mg/d) 2.9 mg/kg/d	96[d]	3.2, (3.2)[e]		

continued over

Table 5.5 continued

Antipsychotics					
Haloperidol	10 mg/d	3.5[b]	2.4%	Infant dose minimal; no untoward effects noted; caution recommended	146,147
	29 mg/d	0.75[b]	0.2%		
Lithium	15 mmol/d	0.12 mmol/kg/d	56%	Severe sedation in some infants. Monitoring of milk and/or infant serum concentrations mandatory. Plasma levels in infants vary from 0.5 to 1/3 of maternal levels 2 weeks postpartum	149,150
Risperidone	6 mg/d	0.8[d]	0.84 (3.5)[e]	Single case. No infant data. Use not recommended until more data available	151
Benzodiazepines					
Diazepam	30 mg/d	13.1[b]	3.0	Some sedation has been reported, but minimal. Acute or occasional use acceptable. Observe for sedation. Depending on dose, avoid prolonged exposure	152,153
	30 mg/d	11.7[b]	2.7 (4.5)[e]		
Lorazepam	5 mg/d	1.8[b]	2.5%	Infant dose low; no untoward effects noted in any breastfeeding infants. Observe for sedation	154,155
	3.5 mg/d	1.35[b]	2.8%		
Midazolam	15	1.4[b]	0.6%	Milk levels are low; no sedation noted in infants. Safe to breastfeed after single doses or short courses	156
Temazepam	10–20 mg/d	Undetectable	No data	Milk concentrations in 9 mothers were extermely low. Depending on dose should be relatively safe	5

[a], safe: term is relative and infants must always be observed closely; [b], calculated from C_{max}; [c], calculated from random timing; [d], calculated from average concentration over dose interval; [e], includes active metabolite

a prospective study of 42 women ingesting sedatives while breastfeeding, there were only three reports of slight infant sedation[162].

Lorazepam has a short half-life (12 h), no active metabolites, and is reported to produce lower cord blood concentrations in newborn infants[154]. When administered in single doses as premedication (3.5 mg orally) 2 h prior to surgery, an average M/P of 0.21 was reported, and milk concentrations were only 8–9 μg/l, which is too low to be clinically relevant[155]. Although other studies showed somewhat higher milk concentrations (23–82 μg/l), these were still too low to produce neurobehavorial changes in newborns[159]. These studies also suggest that neonates are able to metabolize and excrete lorazepam at rates similar to those for adults.

Midazolam, with a short plasma half-life of only 1.9 h, is preferred for rapid induction and maintenance of anesthesia. After oral administration of 15 mg for up to 6 days postnatal, the mean M/P ratio was only 0.15 and the maximum concentration of midazolam in breast milk was 9 μg/l[156]. Midazolam and its 4-hydroxy-metabolite were undetectable in breast milk at 4 h after administration. Thus, the amount of midazolam transferred to an infant via milk is minimal, particularly if the baby is breastfed more than 4 h after administration.

5.8.2 Antipsychotics

The literature covering the antipsychotic medications is very limited. The phenothiazines and thiozanthines transfer into milk in small amounts[163,164]. However their low clearance could predispose the infant to accumulation over time. While only moderate sedation has been reported[163], the use of phenothiazines in neonates has been shown to significantly increase sleep apnea[165], and a relationship with sudden infant death syndrome has been suggested[165–167].

Milk concentrations of haloperidol are low and sedation has not been noted in breastfed infants[147,148,168]. Concentrations of haloperidol in the adult range were found in plasma from two of five infants but there was no evidence of any acute or delayed adverse effects[169]. Three other breastfed infants whose mothers were prescribed both haloperidol and chlorpromazine showed a decline in their developmental scores from the first to the second assessment at 12–18 months[169]. Risperidone has been studied in one patient receiving 6 mg/day[151]. The estimated daily dose of risperidone and metabolites was 4.3% of the weight-adjusted maternal dose.

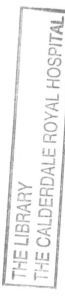

Overall, the use of antipsychotics in breastfeeding women should be approached with caution. Firstly, there are no data about the possible long-term effects on cognitive development. Secondly, an increased incidence of sleep apnea, and possibly of sudden infant death syndrome, suggests that their use should be avoided, particularly in newborns and very young infants[165–167].

5.8.3 Antidepressants

With the introduction of the newer antidepressants, the number of patients receiving treatment for depression has risen markedly. At present, about 10–15% of postpartum women experience clinical depression, although about 80% experience postpartum blues[170]. The consequences to the infant of not treating postpartum depression generally outweigh the hazards of using antidepressants.

In the past the use of antidepressants has been controversial. However, recent evidence that depression itself may interfere with optimal parenting, and that infants of depressed women may suffer from developmental problems, has increased the enthusiasm for early drug treatment of postnatal depression. Children of depressed mothers show more emotional and behavioral disturbances, as well as a delay in expressive language development[171–175]. In general depressed mothers were less responsive to their children and less able to sustain social interaction. Their children were more often distressed, and there was a large variation in quality of mother–child interaction within the depressed group. Thus, it has become important for the clinician to recognize postnatal depression and institute therapy promptly, as the risk of 'not treating' probably outweighs the possible side-effects of drug therapy.

The older tricyclic antidepressants (including amitriptyline, imipramine, desipramine and others), generally show very low transfer into breast milk. With the exception of a single adverse case report on doxepin, Wisner's review of over 29 breastfeeding mother–infant pairs found no detectable drug concentrations in nursling serum, and no reports of adverse effects in breastfed infants[176]. Neurobehavioral development of the breastfed infant exposed to the tricyclic antidepressant dothiepin appears normal[177].

At present, the most popular antidepressants are the serotonin reuptake inhibitors (SSRIs; e.g. citalopram, fluoxetine, fluvoxamine, paroxetine and sertraline) and serotonin–norepinephrine reuptake inhibitors (SNRIs; e.g. venlafaxine). Fluoxetine is of some concern as it is metabolized to norfluoxetine, an active metabolite with a very long half-life of up to 16 days[178,179]. Norfluoxetine has been found in high concentrations in the plasma of several breastfed infants and has been associated with a number of untoward effects such as colic, prolonged crying, increased vomiting, decreased sleep, watery stools, seizures[180,181] and coma (TW Hale, personal communication). The relative infant dose of fluoxetine (plus norfluoxetine) via milk has been reported to be approximately 6.8% (range 2.2–12%) of the maternal dose[135]. It is also known that infants born to mothers who took fluoxetine during their pregnancy have cord plasma concentrations of fluoxetine and norfluoxetine that are similar to those in the mother (Proud S, Rampono J, Ilett KF, unpublished data). In such cases, it is possible that the small amount transferred in breast milk subsequently may augment the concentrations acquired during pregnancy and lead to adverse events, particularly in premature infants. Because concentrations of norfluoxetine were highest in young infants of women ingesting fluoxetine during pregnancy[135], fluoxetine should be used cautiously in patients who are breastfeeding newborn infants, particularly those mothers who used it prenatally. Recent studies have also suggested that fluoxetine used postnatally may reduce weight gain significantly (by 392 g at 6 months of age) in breastfed infants[182].

By contrast, the use of sertraline has been reported in more than 23 mother–infant pairs, and the data show an acceptably low relative infant dose[143,144,183,184]. Plasma concentrations in most infants have been close to, or below, the limit of detection with no reports of untoward effects in the infant. At present, more than 27 mother–infant pairs have been studied while using paroxetine. Milk concentrations have been very low and in most cases paroxetine was not detected in the infant's plasma[141,142,185,186]. At this time, sertraline and paroxetine are probably the SSRIs of first choice for breastfeeding mothers. In a recent study of seven breastfeeding women, the use of citalopram was associated with a relative infant dose of 3.2–3.7%, and no adverse effects were noted[134].

The serotonin and norepinephrine uptake blocker venlafaxine has now been studied in nine lactating mothers[145,146]. Venlafaxine is subject to the cytochrome P4502D6 (CYP2D6) polymorphism in its conversion to its active metabolite O-desmethylvenlafaxine[187,188], which has approximately equal pharmacologic activity[189]. Milk and plasma concentration–time data for two patients are shown in Figure 5.5. These data illustrate the extremes of variability in drug concentration that arise mainly because of CYP2D6 phenotype. Nevertheless, venlafaxine and O-desmethylvenlafaxine have

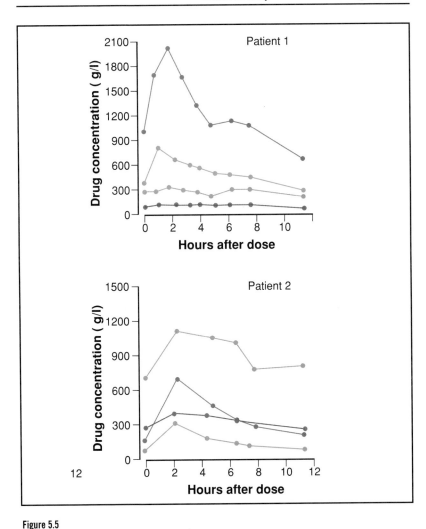

Figure 5.5

Concentration-time profiles for venlafaxine (plasma, ●; milk, ●) and *O*-desmethylvenlafaxine (plasma, ●; milk, ●) in two patients over a dose interval during repeated dose administration. Patient 1 probably has the CYP2D6 poor metabolizer phenotype while patient 2 probably has the CYP2D6 extensive metabolizer phenotype. Figure reproduced with permission from Blackwell Science Publishers, Oxford, UK from Ilett KF, Kristensen JH, Hackett LP, *et al*. Distribution of venlafaxine and its O-desmethyl metabolite in human milk and their effects on breastfed infants. *Br J Clin Pharmacol* 2001;in press

similar pharmacologic activity, and hence the infant exposure can be considered in venlafaxine equivalents. For the nine patients, mean ($\pm$ 95% CI) relative infant doses were 3.3% (2.4–4.3%) for venlafaxine, 3.6% (2.5–4.7%) for O-desmethyl-venlafaxine (as venlafaxine equivalents) and the overall relative infant dose was 6.8% (5.6–8%). Moreover, no adverse effects were noted in their infants despite maternal doses of up to 8.2 mg/kg/d, and measureable levels of O-desmethylvenlafaxine in the plasma of seven of the nine infants.

5.8.4 Lithium

The use of lithium in breastfeeding women has long been controversial. Lithium is a potent medication used to reduce manic symptoms in bipolar disorder, and is known to transfer into human milk in moderate concentrations[149,190,191]. One report of side-effects in a breastfeeding infant included cyanosis, T-wave abnormalities and decreased muscle tone[191]. Most studies suggest that plasma lithium concentrations in breastfed infants are approximately 30–40% of those in the maternal plasma[190-192]. From these studies it is apparent that lithium can distribute into milk and is absorbed by the breastfed infant. Extreme caution is suggested. If the infant continues to breastfeed, close monitoring of lithium concentrations in both infant and mother is recommended. Dehydration is a serious risk and may dramatically increase lithium plasma levels in the infant. Llewellyn and colleagues have published a comprehensive review the use of lithium in pregnancy and lactation[149].

5.9 Radiopharmaceuticals

The use of radioactive substances for diagnostic procedures is quite common in breastfeeding mothers. In some instances, their transfer into milk can be significant and must be closely evaluated to assess the risk. Breastfeeding need not always be discontinued, but in some cases the hazards can be significant. Most often, the mother may need only to withhold breastfeeding for a short interval. However, in some cases (e,g, iodine-131, which is concentrated in the infant thyroid) complete cessation of breastfeeding may be required[194]. The most comprehensive source of information (see Table 5.6) on breastfeeding and radio-pharmaceuticals is published by the Nuclear Regulatory Commission of the United States[195].

5.9.1 Radiocontrast agents

Radiocontrast or radio-opaque agents are opaque to X-rays, and are used to visualize blood vessels in various tissues. Barium sulfate was one of the original agents used, while organic iodinated compounds are used primarily in computed axial tomography and for various X-ray procedures. While iodinated products in general are contraindicated in breastfeeding mothers because of the high milk transfer of iodine, in these products the iodine is covalently bound to the organic molecule and is metabolically stable and virtually not bioavailable. These organic radiocontrast agents are generally rapidly excreted without significant metabolism and the amount of elemental iodine released is minimal. Virtually all of these agents have very short plasma

Table 5.6 Nuclear Regulatory Commission guidelines on discontinuing breastfeeding following the use of radioisotopes* (*Adapted from Nuclear Regulatory Commission Guideline 8.39[2.95])

Radiopharmaceutical	Activity above which instructions are required		Examples of recommended duration of interruption of breastfeeding*
	MBq	mCi	
I-131 NaI	0.01	0.0004	Complete cessation (for this infant or child)
I-123 NaI	20	0.5	
I-123 OIH	100	4	
I-123 mIBG	70	2	24 h for 370 MBq (10 mCi)
			12 h for 150 MBq (4 mCi)
I-125 OIH	3	0.08	
I-131 OIH	10	0.30	
Tc-99m DTPA	1000	30	
Tc-99m MAA	50	1.3	12.6 h for 150 MBq (4 mCi)
Tc-99m Pertechnetate	100	3	24 h for 1100 MBq (30 mCi)
			12 h for 440 MBq (12 mCi)
Tc-99m DISIDA	1000	30	
Tc-99m Glucoheptonate	1000	30	
Tc-99m HAM	400	10	
Tc-99m MIBI	1000	30	
Tc-99m MDP	1000	30	
Tc-99m PYP	900	25	
Tc-99m red blood cell *in vivo* labeling	400	10	6 h for 740 MBq (20 mCi)

continued over

Figure 5.6 continued

Tc-99m red blood cell *in vivo* labeling	1000	30	
Tc-99m sulphur colloid	300	7	6 h for 440 MBq (12 mCi)
Tc-99m DTPA aerosol	1,000	30	
Tc-99m MAG3	1,000	30	
Tc-99m white blood cells	100	4	24 h for 1100 MBq (5 mCi) / 12 h for 440 MBq (2 mCi)
Ga-67 Citrate	1	0.04	1 month for 150 MBq (4 mCi) / 2 weeks for 50 MBq (1.3 mCi) / 1 week for 7 MBq (0.2 mCi)
In-111 white blood cells	10	0.2	1 week for 20 MBq (0.5 mCi)
T1-201 chloride	40	1	2 weeks for 110 MBq (3 mCi)

* The duration of interruption of breastfeeding is selected to reduce the maximum dose to a newborn infant to less than 1 millisievert (0.1 rem), although the regulatory limit is 5 millisieverts (0.5 rem). The actual doses that would be received by most infants would be far below 1 millisievert (0.1 rem). Of course, the physician may use discretion in the recommendation, increasing or decreasing the duration of the interruption.

NOTES: Activities are rounded to one significant figure, except when it was considered appropriate to use two significant figures. Details of the calculations are shown in NUREG-1492, A Regulatory Analysis on Criteria for the Release of Patients Administered Radioactive Material@ (Ref.2).

If there is no recommendation in Column 3 of this table, the maximum activity normally administered is below the activities that require instructions on interruption or discontinuation of breastfeeding half-lives (< 1 h) and, in those studied, milk concentrations were extremely low (Table 5.7). In addition, exposure would be expected to be further decreased because of a low oral bioavailability in the breastfed infant.

Magnetic resonance imaging requires the use of non-iodinated formulations containing the gadolinium ion. These products are very different from the iodinated products. Of the two most common agents used and studied, gadopentetate and gadoteridol, milk levels of gadopentetate were very low[196]. Only 0.023% of the maternal dose was excreted into milk over 24 h. Moreover, the oral bioavailability of gadopentetate in adults is only about 0.8%.

Table 5.7 Radiocontrast agents and their reported milk concentrations

Drug	Dose	Milk (C$_{max}$)	Clinical significance	Bioavailability	References
Gadopentetate	6.5 g	3.09 μmol/l	Only 0.023% of maternal dose; total dose = 0.013μmol/24h; safe	0.8%	196
Iohexol	0.755 g/kg	35 mg/l	Mean milk level was only 11.4 mg/l; virtually unabsorbed; safe	$< 0.1\%$	197
Iopanoic acid	2.77 g	20.8 mg/ 19–29 h	Only 0.08% of maternal dose; virtually unabsorbed; safe	Nil	198
Metrizamide	5.06 g	32.9 mg/l	Only 0.02%of maternal dose; recovered over 44.3 h; poor oral absorption; safe	0.4%	199
Metrizoate	580 mg	14 mg/l	Mean milk level 11.4 mg/24 h; only 0.3% of maternal dose; safe	Nil	197

Apart from the possibility of rare allergic complications, the radiocontrast agents are probably safe to use in breastfeeding mothers. A single pumping and discarding of milk following the procedure could be recommended, but may not be necessary because of the very low bioavailability of these agents.

5.10 Social drugs

Breastfeeding while using drugs of abuse or social drugs is never recommended. However, interruption of breastfeeding following ingestion can be recommended to avoid infant exposure. Table 5.8 provides recommendations for waiting periods following the use of drugs of abuse. These recommendations have been derived empirically from an evaluation of half-life, dose transferred via milk and the overall toxicity of the drug. Large doses of individual medications may require a lengthening

Table 5.8 Recommended duration for interruption of breastfeeding following the last use of social drugs

Drug	Suggested time for discontinuation of breastfeeding
Cocaine	24 h
Amphetamines	24–36 h
Barbiturates	48 h
Phencyclidine	1–2 weeks
LSD	48 h
Ethanol	1 h per drink, or until sober
Heroin	24 h
Marihuana	24 h

of these withholding periods. Chronic abusers should be advised to discontinue breastfeeding.

5.10.1 Alcohol

Alcohol in the blood rapidly equilibrates with milk, and milk concentrations are similar to those in plasma. However, it is interesting that lactating women seem to metabolize ethanol more rapidly than non-lactating women[200]. Nevertheless, unless the mother ingests significant quantities of alcohol, concentrations of ethanol in milk are seldom high enough to produce marked sedation in the infant. Interestingly, alcohol may alter the odor of breast milk, and a 23% decrease in milk production has been noted in some mothers[201]. While the use of alcohol should never be encouraged, the ingestion of one or two small drinks by mothers should not be a major concern. In mothers who ingest large amounts of alcohol, a brief withholding period of 1–2 h per drink should be recommended.

5.10.2 Stimulants

These drugs may cause significant adverse effects in breastfeeding infants and generally, if possible, their use should be avoided. Amphetamine readily transfers into human milk, with an M/P ranging from 3 to 7[202]. However, the data are limited and in this study milk concentrations of amphetamine of 55–138 μg/l were reported. With usual doses of around 15–20 mg/d, the relative infant dose could be as high as 10%. The recreational use of amphetamines is a difficult problem to assess as the dose is not known. A strategy of withholding breastfeeding for 24–36 h would possibly be appropriate in such cases.

While cocaine is quite lipid soluble and in theory should transfer readily into milk, there are minimal data on this drug's entry into milk. However, there is a single case report of acute adverse effects in a breastfed infant whose mother took an unknown quantity of cocaine[203]. Benzoylecgonine, the inactive metabolite of cocaine, will appear in milk for several days following the use of cocaine and the mother should be warned that her infant may test positive for cocaine (actually its metabolite) for a week or more.

5.10.3 Marihuana

Low to moderate concentrations of marihuana have been documented in breast milk[204]. While there are concerns that marihuana may produce dose-dependent sedation and growth delay, in one study of 27 women who smoked marihuana during breastfeeding, no differences were noted in outcomes for infant growth and mental or motor development[205]. Studies in non-lactating women suggest that marihuana can significantly inhibit prolactin secretion[206]. Whether or not this would affect milk production in lactating women is unknown. Infants exposed to marihuana via breast milk may test positive in urine screens for periods of 2–3 weeks[205].

5.10.4 Nicotine

It is estimated that 25% of women in the USA continue to smoke during pregnancy and approximately 8–35% of mothers continue to smoke while breastfeeding[207–209]. Smoking during breastfeeding appears to decrease milk production, fat content, alter the odor and flavor of milk[210], and significantly reduce the overall duration of breastfeeding[211,212]. Nevertheless, millions of mothers have continued to smoke and have breastfed apparently healthy infants worldwide. Nicotine is rapidly transferred into milk and M/P partition ratios of 2:3 have been reported[207,208,213]. Cotinine, the major metabolite of nicotine, is present in the plasma at concentrations that are about 10 times higher than those of nicotine[214], but its nicotinic pharmacologic activity is lower[215]. Although cotinine has cardiovascular and endocrine effects of its own, its M/P transfer ratio is only 0.8[208]. Women should be advised against smoking but, if not able to quit, they should reduce the number of cigarettes smoked as much as possible. The use of nicotine gum and nicotine patches has not been studied in breastfeeding women, but may offer a suitable alternative, as the plasma concentrations of nicotine are reportedly lower than for an equivalent number of cigarettes smoked.

References

1. Weibert RT, Townsend RJ, Kaiser DG, et al. Lack of ibuprofen secretion into human milk. Clin Pharm 1982;1:457–8

2. Townsend RJ, Benedetti TJ, Erickson SH, et al. Excretion of ibuprofen into breast milk. Am J Obstet Gynecol 1984;149:184–6

3. Wischnik A, Manth SM, Lloyd J, et al. The excretion of ketorolac tromethamine into breast milk after multiple oral dosing. Eur J Clin Pharmacol 1989;36(5):521–4

4. Jamali F, Stevens DR. Naproxen excretion in milk and its uptake by the infant [letter]. Drug Intell Clin Pharm 1983;17:910–11

5. Lebedevs TH, Wojnar-Horton RE, Yapp P, et al. Excretion of indomethacin in breast milk. Br J Clin Pharmacol 1991;32:751–4

6. Wittels B, Scott DT, Sinatra RS. Exogenous opioids in human breast milk and acute neonatal neurobehavior: a preliminary study. Anesthesiology 1990;73(5):864–9

7. Feilberg VL, Rosenborg D, Broen CC, et al. Excretion of morphine in human breast milk. Acta Anaesthesiol Scand 1989;33(5):426–8

8. Wojnar-Horton RE, Kristensen JH, Yapp P, et al. Methadone distribution and excretion into breast milk of clients in a methadone maintenance programme. Br J Clin Pharmacol 1997;44(6):543–7

9. Begg EJ, Malpas TJ, Hackett LP, et al. Distribution of R- and S-methadone into human milk at steady state during ingestion of medium to high doses. Br J Clin Pharmacol 2001;in press

10. Geraghty B, Graham EA, Logan B, et al. Methadone levels in breast milk. J Human Lact 1997;13(3):227–30

11. Peiker G, Muller B, Ihn W, et al. Excretion of pethidine in mother's milk [in German]. Zentralbl Gynakol 1980;102:537–41

12. Quinn PG, Kuhnert BR, Kaine CJ, et al. Measurement of meperidine and normeperidine in human breast milk by selected ion monitoring. Biomed Environ Mass Spectrom 1986;13:133–5

13. Leuschen MP, Wolf LJ, Rayburn WF. Fentanyl excretion in breast milk [letter]. Clin Pharm 1990;9:336–7

14. Madej TH, Strunin L. Comparison of epidural fentanyl with sufentanil. Analgesia and side-effects after a single bolus dose during elective caesarean section. Anaesthesia 1987;42(11):1156–61

15. Figalgo I. Anemia aguda, rectaorragia y hematuria asociadas a la ingestion de naproxen. Anales Españoles Pediatr 1989;30:317–19

16. Eeg-Olofsson O, Malmros I, Elwin CE, et al. Convulsions in a breast-fed infant after maternal indomethacin [letter]. Lancet 1978;2:215

17. Blinick G, Inturrisi CE, Jerez E, et al. Methadone assays in pregnant women and progeny. Am J Obstet Gynecol 1975;121:617–21

18. Pond SM, Kreek MJ, Tong TG, et al. Altered methadone pharmacokinetics in methadone-maintained pregnant women. J Pharmacol Exp Ther 1985;233:1–6

19. McCarthy JJ, Posey BL. Methadone levels in human milk. J Human Lact 2000;16:115–20

20. Kristensen K, Blemmer T, Angelo HR, et al. Stereoselective pharmacokinetics of methadone in chronic pain patients. Ther Drug Monit 1996;18:221–7

21. Codd EE, Shank RP, Schupsky JJ, et al. Serotonin and norepinephrine uptake inhibiting activity of centrally acting analgesics: structural determinants and role in antinociception. J Pharmacol Exp Ther 1995;274:1263–70

22. Ebert B, Thorkildsen C, Andersen S, et al. Opioid analgesics as noncompetitive N-methyl-D-aspartate (NMDA) antagonists [Review]. Biochem Pharmacol 1998;56:553–9

23. White JM, Irvine RJ. Future directions in opioid overdose. Addiction 1999;94:978–80

24. Eap CB, Cuendet C, Baumann P. Binding of d-methadone, l-methadone, and dl-methadone to proteins in plasma of healthy volunteers: role of the variants of alpha 1-acid glycoprotein. Clin Pharmacol Ther 1990;47:338–46

25. Ostrea EM, Chavez CJ, Strauss ME. A study of factors that influence the severity of neonatal narcotic withdrawal. J Pediatr

1976;88:642–5

26.   Newman RG, Bashkow S, Calko D. Results of 313 consecutive live births of infants delivered to patients in the New York City Methadone Maintenance Treatment Program. *Am J Obstet Gynecol* 1975;121:233–7

27.   Strauss ME, Andresko M, Stryker JC, *et al*. Methadone maintenance during pregnancy: pregnancy, birth, and neonate characteristics. *Am J Obstet Gynecol* 1974;120:895–900

28.   Malpas TJ, Darlow BA, Lennox R, *et al*. Maternal methadone dosage and neonatal withdrawal. *Aust NZ J Obstet Gynaecol* 1995;35:175–7

29.   Malpas TJ, Darlow BA. Neonatal abstinence syndrome following abrupt cessation of breastfeeding. *NZ Med J* 1999;112:12–13

30.   Smialek JE, Monforte JR, Aronow R, *et al*. Methadone deaths in children. A continuing problem. *JAMA* 1977;238:2516–17

31.   Terwilliger WG, Hatcher RA. The elimination of morphine and quinine in human milk. *Surg Gynecol Obstet* 1934;58:823–6

32.   Kwit NT, Hatcher RA. Excretion of drugs in milk. *Am J Dis Child* 1935;49:900–4

33.   Robieux I, Koren G, Vandenbergh H, *et al*. Morphine excretion in breast milk and resultant exposure of a nursing infant. *J Toxicol Clin Toxicol* 1990;28:365–70

34.   Pynnonen S, Kanto J, Sillanpaa M, *et al*. Carbamazepine: placental transport, tissue concentrations in foetus and newborn, and level in milk. *Acta Pharmacol Toxicol (Copenh)* 1977;41:244–53

35.   Niebyl JR, Blake DA, Freeman JM, *et al*. Carbamazepine levels in pregnancy and lactation. *Obstet Gynecol* 1979;53:139–40

36.   Ohman I, Vitols S, Tomson T. Lamotrigine in pregnancy: pharmacokinetics during delivery, in the neonate, and during lactation. *Epilepsia* 2000;41:709–13

37.   Tomson T, Ohman I, Vitols S. Lamotrigine in pregnancy and lactation: a case report. *Epilepsia* 1997;38:1039–41

38.   Rambeck B, Kurlemann G, Stodieck SR, *et al*. Concentrations of lamotrigine in a mother on lamotrigine treatment and her newborn child. *Eur J Clin Pharmacol* 1997;51:481–4

39.   Cruikshank DP, Varner MW, Pitkin RM. Breast milk magnesium and calcium concentrations following magnesium sulfate treatment. *Am J Obstet Gynecol* 1982;143: 685–8

40.   Nau H, Kuhnz W, Egger HJ, *et al*. Anticonvulsants during pregnancy and lactation. Transplacental, maternal and neonatal pharmacokinetics. *Clin Pharmacokinet* 1982;7:508–43

41.   Steen B, Rane A, Lonnerholm G, *et al*. Phenytoin excretion in human breast milk and plasma levels in nursed infants. *Ther Drug Monit* 1982;4:331–4

42.   von Unruh GE, Froescher W, Hoffmann F, *et al*. Valproic acid in breast milk: how much is really there? *Ther Drug Monit* 1984;6:272–6

43.   Nau H, Rating D, Koch S, *et al*. Valproic acid and its metabolites: placental transfer, neonatal pharmacokinetics, transfer via mother's milk and clinical status in neonates of epileptic mothers. *J Pharmacol Exp Ther* 1981;219:768–77

44.   Juul S. Barbiturate poisoning via breast milk? *Ugeskr Laeger* 1969;131:2257–8

45.   Kaneko S, Sato T, Suzuki K. The levels of anticonvulsants in breast milk. *Br J Clin Pharmacol* 1979;7:624–7

46.   Johannessen SI. Pharmacokinetics of valproate in pregnancy: mother–foetus–newborn. *Pharm Weekbl Sci* 1992;14:114–17

47.   Dooley J, Camfield P, Gordon K, et al. Lamotrigine-induced rash in children. *Neurology* 1996;46:240–2

48.   Hilbert J. Excretion of loratadine in human breast milk. *J Clin Pharmacol* 1988;28:234–9

49.   Lucas BD, Purdy CY, Scarim SK, *et al*. Terfenadine pharmacokinetics in breast milk in lactating women. *Clin Pharmacol Ther* 1995;57:398–402

50.   Peiker G, Schroder S. Investigations concerning concentrations of oxacillin and ampicillin in the serum of mothers suffering from mastitis puerperalis. *Pharmazie* 1986;41:793–5

51. Kafetzis DA, Siafas CA, Georgakopoulos PA, et al. Passage of cephalosporins and amoxicillin into the breast milk. *Acta Paediatr Scand* 1981;70:285–8

52. Matsuda S. Transfer of antibiotics into maternal milk. *Biol Res Pregnancy Perinatol* 1984;5:57–60

53. McEvoy GE, ed. *AHFS Drug Information*, 1995

54. Yoshioka H, Cho K, Takimoto M, et al. Transfer of cefazolin into human milk. *J Pediatr* 1979;94:151–2

55. Kafetzis DA, Lazarides CV, Siafas CA, et al. Transfer of cefotaxime in human milk and from mother to foetus. *J Antimicrob Chemother* 1980;6 (suppl A):135–41

56. Roex AJ, van Loenen AC, Puyenbroek JI, et al. Secretion of cefoxitin in breast milk following short-term prophylactic administration in caesarean section. *Eur J Obstet Gynecol Reprod Biol* 1987;25:299–302

57. Blanco JD, Jorgensen JH, Castaneda YS, et al. Ceftazidime levels in human breast milk. *Antimicrob Agents Chemother* 1983;23:479–80

58. Celiloglu M, Celiker S, Guven H, et al. Gentamicin excretion and uptake from breast milk by nursing infants. *Obstet Gynecol* 1994;84:263–5

59. Snider DEJ, Powell KE. Should women taking antituberculosis drugs breast-feed? *Arch Intern Med* 1984;144:589–90

60. Knowles JA. Drugs in milk. *Pediatr Currents* 1972;1:28–32

61. Kelsey JJ, Moser LR, Jennings JC, et al. Presence of azithromycin breast milk concentrations: a case report. *Am J Obstet Gynecol* 1994;170:1375–6

62. Giamarellou H, Kolokythas E, Petrikkos G, et al. Pharmacokinetics of three newer quinolones in pregnant and lactating women. *Am J Med* 1989;87:49s–51s

63. Gardner DK, Gabbe SG, Harter C. Simultaneous concentrations of ciprofloxacin in breast milk and in serum in mother and breast-fed infant. *Clin Pharm* 1992;11:352–4

64. Harmon T, Burkhart G, Applebaum H. Perforated pseudomembranous colitis in the breast-fed infant. *J Pediatr Surg* 1992;27: 744–6

65. Meyer LJ, de Miranda P, Sheth N, et al. Acyclovir in human breast milk. *Am J Obstet Gynecol* 1988;158:586–8

66. Taddio A, Klein J, Koren G. Acyclovir excretion in human breast milk. *Ann Pharmacother* 1994;28:585–7

67. Mann CF. Clindamycin and breast-feeding [letter]. *Pediatrics* 1980;66:1030–1

68. Smith JA, Morgan JR. Clindamycin in human breastmilk. *Can Med Ass J* 1975;112:806

69. Morganti G, Ceccarelli G, Ciaffi G. Comparative concentrations of a tetracycline antibiotic in serum and maternal milk. *Antibiotica* 1968;6:216–23

70. Force RW. Fluconazole concentrations in breast milk. *Pediatr Infect Dis J* 1995;14:235–6

71. Passmore CM, McElnay JC, Rainey EA, et al. Metronidazole excretion in human milk and its effect on the suckling neonate. *Br J Clin Pharmacol* 1988;26:45–51

72. Heisterberg L, Branebjerg PE. Blood and milk concentrations of metronidazole in mothers and infants. *J Perinat Med* 1983;11:114–20

73. Erickson SH, Oppenheim GL, Smith GH. Metronidazole in breast milk. *Obstet Gynecol* 1981;57:48–50

74. Hosbach RH, Foster RB. Absence of nitrofurantoin from human milk. *JAMA* 1967;202:1057

75. Varsano I, Fischl J, Shochet SB. The excretion of orally ingested nitrofurantoin in human milk. *J Pediatr* 1973;82:886–7

76. Lenzi E, Santuari S. Preliminary observations on the use of a new semi-synthetic rifamycin derivative in gynecology and obstetrics. *Atti Accad Lancisiana Roma* 1969;13 (suppl 1):87–94

77. Posner AC, Prigot A, Konicoff NG. *Medical Encyclopedia, Antibiotics Annual*. New York, 1955:594

78. Reyes MP, Ostrea EMJ, Cabinian AE, et

al. Vancomycin during pregnancy: does it cause hearing loss or nephrotoxicity in the infant? *Am J Obstet Gynecol* 1989;161:977–81

79.   Sanders CC. Cefepime: the next generation? *Clin Infect Dis* 1993;17:369–79

80.   Shyu WC, Shah VR, Campbell DA, et al. Excretion of cefprozil into human breast milk. *Antimicrob Agents Chemother* 1992;36:938–41

81.   Mischler TW, Corson SL, Larranaga A, et al. Cephradine and epicillin in body fluids of lactating and pregnant women. *J Reprod Med* 1978;21:130–6

82.   Bennett PN. *Drugs and Human Lactation*, 2nd edn. Amsterdam: Elsevier, 1996:192–3

83.   Amir LH, Garland SM, Dennerstein L, et al. *Candida albicans*: is it associated with nipple pain in lactating women? *Gynecol Obstet Invest* 1996;41:30–4

84.   Blaschke-Hellmessen R, Henker J, Futschik M. Results of mycologic studies of donated breast milk. *Kinderarztl Prax* 1991;59:77–80

85.   Vudhichamnong K, Walker DM, Ryley HC. The effect of secretory immunoglobulin A on the *in-vitro* adherence of the yeast *Candida albicans* to human oral epithelial cells. *Arch Oral Biol* 1982;27:617–21

86.   Livingston V, Stringer J. The treatment of Staphyloccocus aureus infected sore nipples: a randomized comparative study. *J Human Lact* 1999;15:241–6

87.   The Harriet Lane Service Children's Medical and Surgical Center of the Johns Hopkins Hospital. In: Siberry GK, Iannone R, eds. *The Harriet Lane Handbook: a Manual for Pediatric House Officers*, 15th edn. St Louis: Mosby, 2000:717

88.   Kauffman RE, O'Brien C, Gilford P. Sulfisoxazole secretion into human milk. *J Pediatr* 1980;97:839–41

89.   Louis A, Pagliaro AMP, eds. *Problems in pediatric drug therapy*, 2nd edn. Hamilton, IL: Drug Intelligence Publications, 1987

90.   Cover DL, Mueller BA. Ciprofloxacin penetration into human breast milk: a case report. *DICP* 1990;24:703–4

91.   Earl P, Sisson PR, Ingham HR. Twelve-hourly dosage schedule for oral and intravenous metronidazole. *J Antimicrob Chemother* 1989;23:619–21

92.   Hale TW. *Medications and mothers' milk*, 9th edn. Amarillo, TX: Pharmasoft, 2000:589

93.   Yeager AS. Use of acyclovir in premature and term neonates. *Am J Med* 1982;73:205–9

94.   Benet LZ, Oie S, Schwartz JB. Hardman JG, Limbird LE, eds. *Goodman & Gilman's The Pharmacological Basis of Medicine*, 9th edn. New York: McGraw Hill, 1996:1707–92

95.   Acosta EP, Fletcher CV. Valacyclovir. *Ann Pharmacother* 1997;31:185–91

96.   Boutroy MJ, Bianchetti G, Dubruc C, et al. To nurse when receiving acebutolol: is it dangerous for the neonate? *Eur J Clin Pharmacol* 1986;30:737–9

97.   Thorley KJ, McAinsh J. Levels of the beta-blockers atenolol and propranolol in the breast milk of women treated for hypertension in pregnancy. *Biopharm Drug Dispos* 1983;4:299–301

98.   White WB, Andreoli JW, Wong SH, et al. Atenolol in human plasma and breast milk. *Obstet Gynecol* 1984;63 (3 Suppl):42s–4s

99.   Kulas J, Lunell NO, Rosing U, et al. Atenolol and metoprolol. A comparison of their excretion into human breast milk. *Acta Obstet Gynecol Scand* 1984;118 (suppl):65–9

100.   Lunell NO, Kulas J, Rane A. Transfer of labetalol into amniotic fluid and breast milk in lactating women. *Eur J Clin Pharmacol* 1985;28:597–9

101.   Sandstrom B, Regardh CG. Metoprolol excretion into breast milk. *Br J Clin Pharmacol* 1980;9:518–19

102.   Smith MT, Livingstone I, Hooper WD, et al. Propranolol, propranolol glucuronide, and naphthoxylactic acid in breast milk and plasma. *Ther Drug Monit* 1983;5:87–93

103.   Devlin RG, Fleiss PM. Captopril in human blood and breast milk. *J Clin Pharmacol* 1981;21:110–13

104.   Redman CW, Kelly JG, Cooper WD. The

excretion of enalapril and enalaprilat in human breast milk. *Eur J Clin Pharmacol* 1990;38:99

105. Begg EJ, Robson RA, Gardiner SJ, *et al.* Quinapril and its metabolite quinaprilat in human milk. *Br J Clin Pharmacol* 2001:478–81

106. Okada M, Inoue H, Nakamura Y, *et al.* Excretion of diltiazem in human milk [Letter]. *N Engl J Med* 1985;312:992–3

107. Ehrenkranz RA, Ackerman BA, Hulse JD. Nifedipine transfer into human milk. *J Pediatr* 1989;114:478–80

108. Manninen AK, Juhakoski A. Nifedipine concentrations in maternal and umbilical serum, amniotic fluid, breast milk and urine of mothers and offspring. *Int J Clin Pharmacol Res* 1991;11:231–6

109. Penny WJ, Lewis MJ. Nifedipine is excreted in human milk. *Eur J Clin Pharmacol* 1989;36:427–8

110. Anderson P, Bondesson U, Mattiasson I, *et al.* Verapamil and norverapamil in plasma and breast milk during breast feeding. *Eur J Clin Pharmacol* 1987;31:625–7

111. Inoue H, Unno N, Ou MC, *et al.* Level of verapamil in human milk [Letter]. *Eur J Clin Pharmacol* 1984;26:657–8

112. White WB, Andreoli JW, Cohn RD. Alpha-methyldopa disposition in mothers with hypertension and in their breast-fed infants. *Clin Pharmacol Ther* 1985;37:387–90

113. Jones HM, Cummings AJ. A study of the transfer of alpha-methyldopa to the human foetus and newborn infant. *Br J Clin Pharmacol* 1978;6:432–4

114. Hartikainen-Sorri AL, Heikkinen JE, Koivisto M. Pharmacokinetics of clonidine during pregnancy and nursing. *Obstet Gynecol* 1987;69:598–600

115. Bunjes R, Schaefer C, Holzinger D. Clonidine and breast-feeding [Letter]. *Clin Pharm* 1993;12:178–9

116. Briggs GG, Freeman RK, Yaffee SJ. *Drugs in Pregnancy and Lactation*. Philadelphia: Lippincott Williams & Wilkins, 1998

117. Schimmel MS, Eidelman AI, Wilschanski MA, *et al.* Toxic effects of atenolol consumed

during breast feeding. *J Pediatr* 1989;114:476–8

118. Taylor EA, Turner P. Anti-hypertensive therapy with propranolol during pregnancy and lactation. *Postgrad Med J* 1981;57:427–30

119. Bauer JH, Pape B, Zajicek J, *et al.* Propranolol in human plasma and breast milk. *Am J Cardiol* 1979;43:860–2

120. Liedholm H, Wahlin-Boll E, Hanson A, *et al.* Transplacental passage and breast milk concentrations of hydralazine. *Eur J Clin Pharmacol* 1982;21:417–19

121. Andersen HJ. Excretion of verapamil in human milk. *Eur J Clin Pharmacol* 1983;25:279–80

122. Ost L, Wettrell G, Bjorkhem I, *et al.* Prednisolone excretion in human milk. *J Pediatr* 1985;106:1008–11

123. Berlin CM. Excretion of prednisone and prednisolone in human milk. *The Pharmacologist* 1979;21:264

124. Vree TB, Lagerwerf AJ, Verwey-van Wissen CP, *et al.* High-performance liquid chromatography analysis, preliminary pharmacokinetics, metabolism and renal excretion of methylprednisolone with its C6 and C20 hydroxy metabolites in multiple sclerosis patients receiving high-dose pulse therapy. *J Chromatogr B Biomed Sci Appl* 1999;732:337–48

125. Siberry GK, Iannone R, eds. *The Harriet Lane Handbook: a Manual for Pediatric House Officers*, 15th edn. St Louis: Mosby, 2000:770

126. Mizuta H, Amino N, Ichihara K, *et al.* Thyroid hormones in human milk and their influence on thyroid function of breast-fed babies. *Pediatr Res* 1983;17:468–71

127. Oberkotter LV. Thyroid function and human breast milk [Letter]. *Am J Dis Child* 1983;137:1131

128. Sato T, Suzuki Y. Presence of triiodothyronine, no detectable thyroxine and reverse triiodothyronine in human milk. *Endocrinol Jpn* 1979;26:507–13

129. Kampmann JP, Johansen K, Hansen JM, *et al.* Propylthiouracil in human milk. Revision of

a dogma. *Lancet* 1980;1:736–7

130. Low LC, Lang J, Alexander WD. Excretion of carbimazole and propylthiouracil in breast milk [Letter]. *Lancet* 1979;2:1011

131. Johansen K, Andersen AN, Kampmann JP, *et al.* Excretion of methimazole in human milk. *Eur J Clin Pharmacol* 1982;23:339–41

132. Bennett PN. In: Bennett PN, ed. *Drugs and Human Lactation*, 2nd edn. Amsterdam: Elsevier, 1996:283–4

133. Azizi F, Khoshniat M, Bahrainian M, *et al.* Thyroid function and intellectual development of infants nursed by mothers taking methimazole. *J Clin Endocrinol Metab* 2000;85:3233–8

134. Rampono J, Kristensen JH, Hackett LP, *et al.* Citalopram and demethylcitalopram in human milk; distribution, excretion and effects in breast fed infants. *Br J Clin Pharmacol* 2000;50:263–8

135. Kristensen JH, Ilett KF, Hackett LP, *et al.* Distribution and excretion of fluoxetine and norfluoxetine in human milk. *Br J Clin Pharmacol* 1999;48:521–7

136. Taddio A, Ito S, Koren G. Excretion of fluoxetine and its metabolite, norfluoxetine, in human breast milk. *J Clin Pharmacol* 1996;36:42–7

137. Wright S, Dawling S, Ashford JJ. Excretion of fluvoxamine in breast milk. *Br J Clin Pharmacol* 1991;31:209

138. Yoshida K, Smith B, Channikumar R. Fluvoxamine in breast-milk and infant development. *Br J Clin Pharmacol* 1997;44:210–11

139. Dodd S, Buist A, Burrows GD, *et al.* Determination of nefazodone and its pharmacologically active metabolites in human blood plasma and breast milk by high-performance liquid chromatography. *J Chromatog B: Biomed Appl* 1999;730:249–55

140. Yapp P, Ilett KF, Kristensen JH, *et al.* Drowsiness and poor-feeding in a breast-fed infant: association with nefazodone and its metabolites. *Ann Pharmacother* 2000;34:1269–72

141. Stowe ZN, Cohen LS, Hostetter A, *et al.* Paroxetine in human breast milk and nursing infants. *Am J Psychiatry* 2000;157:185–9

142. Begg EJ, Duffull SB, Saunders DA, *et al.* Paroxetine in human milk. *Br J Clin Pharmacol* 1999;48:142–7

143. Kristensen JH, Ilett KF, Dusci LJ, *et al.* Distribution and excretion of sertraline and N-desmethylsertraline in human milk. *Br J Clin Pharmacol* 1998;45:453–7

144. Stowe ZN, Owens MJ, Landry JC, *et al.* Sertraline and desmethylsertraline in human breast milk and nursing infants. *Am J Psychiatry* 1997;154:1255–60

145. Ilett KF, Hackett LP, Dusci LJ, *et al.* Distribution and excretion of venlafaxine and O-desmethylvenlafaxine in human milk. *Br J Clin Pharmacol* 1998;45:459–62

146. Ilett KF, Kristensen JH, Hackett LP, *et al.* Distribution of venlafaxine and its O-desmethyl metabolite in human milk and their effects on breastfed infants. *Br J Clin Pharmacol* 2001;in press

147. Whalley LJ, Blain PG, Prime JK. Haloperidol secreted in breast milk. *Br Med J* (Clin Res Ed) 1981;282:1746–7

148. Stewart RB, Karas B, Springer PK. Haloperidol excretion in human milk. *Am J Psychiatry* 1980;137:849–50

149. Llewellyn A, Stowe ZN, Strader JRJ. The use of lithium and management of women with bipolar disorder during pregnancy and lactation [Review]. *J Clin Psychiat* 1998;59 (suppl 6):57–64; discussion 65:57–64

150. Schou M, Amdisen A. Lithium and pregnancy. 3. Lithium ingestion by children breast-fed by women on lithium treatment. *Br Med J* 1973;2:138

151. Hill RC, McIvor RJ, Wojnar-Horton RE, *et al.* Risperidone distribution and excretion into human milk: case report and estimated infant exposure during breast-feeding [Letter]. *J Clin Psychopharmacol* 2000;20:285–6

152. Erkkola R, Kanto J. Diazepam and breast-feeding. *Lancet* 1972;1:1235–6

153. Wesson DR, Camber S, Harkey M, *et al.* Diazepam and desmethyldiazepam in breast

milk. *J Psychoactive Drugs* 1985;17:55–6

154. Whitelaw AG, Cummings AJ, McFadyen IR. Effect of maternal lorazepam on the neonate. *Br Med J (Clin Res Ed)* 1981;282:1106–8

155. Summerfield RJ, Nielsen MS. Excretion of lorazepam into breast milk [Letter]. *Br J Anaesth* 1985;57:1042–3

156. Matheson I, Lunde PK, Bredesen JE. Midazolam and nitrazepam in the maternity ward: milk concentrations and clinical effects. *Br J Clin Pharmacol* 1990;30:787–93

157. Cole AP, Hailey DM. Diazepam and active metabolite in breast milk and their transfer to the neonate. *Arch Dis Child* 1975;50:741–2

158. Spigset O. Anaesthetic agents and excretion in breast milk. *Acta Anaesthesiol Scand* 1994;38:94–103

159. McBride RJ, Dundee JW, Moore J, *et al.* A study of the plasma concentrations of lorazepam in mother and neonate. *Br J Anaesth* 1979;51:971–8

160. Fisher JB, Edgren BE, Mammel MC, *et al.* Neonatal apnea associated with maternal clonazepam therapy: a case report. *Obstet Gynecol* 1985;66 (3 Suppl):34s–5s

161. Wretlind M. Excretion of oxazepam in breast milk. *Eur J Clin Pharmacol* 1987;33:209–10

162. Ito S, Blajchman A, Stephenson M, *et al.* Prospective follow-up of adverse reactions in breast-fed infants exposed to maternal medication. *Am J Obstet Gynecol* 1993;168:1393–9

163. Wiles DH, Orr MW, Kolakowska T. Chlorpromazine levels in plasma and milk of nursing mothers [Letter]. *Br J Clin Pharmacol* 1978;5:272–3

164. Blacker KH. Mothers milk and chlorpromazine. *Am J Psychiatry* 1962;114:178–9

165. Kahn A, Hasaerts D, Blum D. Phenothiazine-induced sleep apneas in normal infants. *Pediatrics* 1985;75:844–7

166. Pollard AJ, Rylance G. Inappropriate prescribing of promethazine in infants [Letter]. *Arch Dis Child* 1994;70:357

167. Cantu TG. Phenothiazines and sudden infant death syndrome. *DICP* 1989;23:795–6

168. Ohkubo T, Shimoyama R, Sugawara K. Measurement of haloperidol in human breast milk by high-performance liquid chromatography. *J Pharm Sci* 1992;81:947–9

169. Yoshida K, Smith B, Craggs M, *et al.* Neuroleptic drugs in breast-milk: a study of pharmacokinetics and of possible adverse effects in breast-fed infants. *Psychol Med* 1998;28:81–91

170. O'Hara MW, Zekoski EM, Philipps LH, *et al.* Controlled prospective study of postpartum mood disorders: comparison of childbearing and nonchildbearing women. *J Abnorm Psychol* 1990;99:3–15

171. Zekoski EM, O'Hara MW, Wills KE. The effects of maternal mood on mother-infant interaction. *J Abnorm Child Psychol* 1987;15:361–78

172. Sinclair D, Murray L. Effects of postnatal depression on children's adjustment to school. Teacher's reports. *Br J Psychiatry* 1998;172:58–63

173. Lee CM, Gotlib IH. Adjustment of children of depressed mothers: a 10-month follow-up. *J Abnorm Psychol* 1991;100:473–7

174. Murray L, Fiori-Cowley A, Hooper R, *et al.* The impact of postnatal depression and associated adversity on early mother–infant interactions and later infant outcome. *Child Dev* 1996;67:2512–26

175. Lovejoy MC. Maternal depression: effects on social cognition and behavior in parent–child interactions. *J Abnorm Child Psychol* 1991;19:693–706

176. Wisner KL, Perel JM, Findling RL. Antidepressant treatment during breast-feeding. *Am J Psychiatry* 1996;153:1132–7

177. Buist A, Janson H. Effect of exposure to dothiepin and northiaden in breast milk on child development. *Br J Psychiatry* 1995;167:370–3

178. Lemberger L, Bergstrom RF, Wolen RL, *et al.* Fluoxetine: clinical pharmacology and physiologic disposition. *J Clin Psychiatry* 1985;46:14–19

179. Nash JF, Bopp RJ, Carmichael RH, et al. Determination of fluoxetine and norfluoxetine in plasma by gas chromatography with electron-capture detection. Clin Chem 1982;28:2100–2

180. Lester BM, Cucca J, Andreozzi L, et al. Possible association between fluoxetine hydrochloride and colic in an infant. J Am Acad Child Adolesc Psychiatry 1993;32:1253–5

181. Spencer MJ. Fluoxetine hydrochloride (Prozac) toxicity in a neonate. Pediatrics 1993;92:721–2

182. Chambers CD, Anderson PO, Thomas RG, et al. Weight gain in infants breastfed by mothers who take fluoxetine. Pediatrics 1999;104:e61

183. Altshuler LL, Burt VK, McMullen M, et al. Breastfeeding and sertraline: a 24-hour analysis. J Clin Psychiatry 1995;56:243–5

184. Mammen OK, Perel JM, Rudolph G, et al. Sertraline and norsertraline levels in three breastfed infants. J Clin Psychiatry 1997;58:100–3

185. Ohman R, Hagg S, Carleborg L, et al. Excretion of paroxetine into breast milk. J Clin Psychiatry 1999;60:519–23

186. Spigset O, Carleborg L, Norstrom A, et al. Paroxetine level in breast milk [Letter]. J Clin Psychiatry 1996;57:39

187. Fukuda T, Nishida Y, Zhou Q, et al. The impact of the CYP2D6 and CYP2C19 genotypes on venlafaxine pharmacokinetics in a Japanese population. Eur J Clin Pharmacol 2000;56:175–80

188. Fukuda T, Yamamoto I, Nishida Y, et al. Effect of the CYP2D6*10 genotype on venlafaxine pharmacokinetics in healthy adult volunteers. Br J Clin Pharmacol 1999;47:450–3

189. Muth EA, Moyer JA, Haskins T, et al. Biochemical, neurophysiological, and behavioural effects of Wy-45,233 and other identified metabolites of the antidepressant venlafaxine. Drug Dev Res 1991;23:191–9

190. Sykes PA, Quarrie J, Alexander FW. Lithium carbonate and breast-feeding. Br Med J 1976;2:1299

191. Tunnessen WWJ, Hertz CG. Toxic effects of lithium in newborn infants: a commentary. J Pediatr 1972;81:804–7

192. Fries H. Lithium in pregnancy. Lancet 1970;1:1233

193. Montgomery A. Use of lithium for treatment of bipolar disorder during pregnancy and lactation. Acad Breastfeeding Med News View 1997;3:4–5

194. Saenz RB. Iodine-131 elimination from breast milk: a case report. J Human Lact 2000;16:44–6

195. U.S. Nuclear Regulatory Commission. Activities of radiopharmaceuticals that require instructions and records when administered to patients who are breast-feeding an infant or child. Regulatory Guide 8.39. Bethesda: U.S.: Nuclear Regulatory Commission, 1999: http://www.nrc.gov/NRC/RG/08/08-039.html

196. Rofsky NM, Weinreb JC, Litt AW. Quantitative analysis of gadopentetate dimeglumine excreted in breast milk. J Magn Reson Imaging 1993;3:131–2

197. Nielsen ST, Matheson I, Rasmussen JN, et al. Excretion of iohexol and metrizoate in human breast milk. Acta Radiol 1987;28:523–6

198. Holmdahl KH. Cholecystography during lactation. Acta Radiol 1956;45:305–7

199. Ilett KF, Hackett LP, Paterson JW, et al. Excretion of metrizamide in milk [Letter]. Br J Radiol 1981;54:537–8

200. da-Silva VA, Malheiros LR, Moraes-Santos AR, et al. Ethanol pharmacokinetics in lactating women. Braz J Med Biol Res 1993;26:1097–103

201. Mennella JA, Beauchamp GK. The transfer of alcohol to human milk. Effects on flavor and the infant's behavior. N Engl J Med 1991;325:981–5

202. Steiner E, Villen T, Hallberg M, et al. Amphetamine secretion in breast milk. Eur J Clin Pharmacol 1984;27:123–4

203. Chasnoff IJ, Lewis DE, Squires L. Cocaine intoxication in a breast-fed infant. Pediatrics 1987;80:836–8

204. Perez-Reyes M, Wall ME. Presence of Δ9-tetrahydrocannabinol in human milk [Letter]. N Engl J Med 1982;307:819–20

205. Tennes K, Avitable N, Blackard C, et al. Marijuana: prenatal and postnatal exposure in the human. *NIDA Res Monogr* 1985;59:48–60

206. Mendelson JH, Mello NK, Ellingboe J. Acute effects of marihuana smoking on prolactin levels in human females. *J Pharmacol Exp Ther* 1985;232:220–2

207. Labrecque M, Marcoux S, Weber JP, et al. Feeding and urine cotinine values in babies whose mothers smoke. *Pediatrics* 1989;83:93–7

208. Luck W, Nau H. Nicotine and cotinine concentrations in serum and milk of nursing smokers. *Br J Clin Pharmacol* 1984;18:9–15

209. Stepans MB, Wilkerson N. Physiologic effects of maternal smoking on breast-feeding infants. *J Am Acad Nurse Practitioners* 1993;5:105–13

210. Vio F, Salazar G, Infante C. Smoking during pregnancy and lactation and its effects on breast-milk volume. *Am J Clin Nutr* 1991;54:1011–16

211. Hopkinson JM, Schanler RJ, Fraley JK, et al. Milk production by mothers of premature infants: influence of cigarette smoking. *Pediatrics* 1992;90:934–8

212. Mennella JA, Beauchamp GK. Smoking and the flavor of breast milk [Letter]. *N Engl J Med* 1998;339:1559–60

213. Luck W, Nau H. Nicotine and cotinine concentrations in the milk of smoking mothers: influence of cigarette consumption and diurnal variation. *Eur J Pediat* 1987;146:21–6

214. Gupta SK, Hwang SS, Causey D, et al. Comparison of the nicotine pharmacokinetics of Nicoderm (nicotine transdermal system) and half-hourly cigarette smoking. *J Clin Pharmacol* 1995;35:985–9

215. Keenan RM, Hatsukami DK, Pentel PR, c. Pharmacodynamic effects of cotinine in abstinent cigarette smokers. *Clin Pharmacol Ther* 1994;55:581–90

Chapter 6
Conclusion

It is well known that the health benefits of breastfeeding are significant, for both the mother and the infant. The reduction of infectious and other diseases in breastfed infants compared with formula-fed infants is now well documented. Nevertheless, the use of medications in breastfeeding mothers is often a divisive question that may cause conflict between the mother, her physician and other healthcare professionals. It is important to note that disrupting breastfeeding, even for a short time, can be detrimental to the mother's milk supply.

While most drugs will transfer into milk, the vast majority do so at concentrations so low that adverse effects in the infant are rare. By understanding the mechanisms by which medications transfer into milk, quantifying the extent of such transfer, identifying truly hazardous medications, and identifying those infants who are most at risk, the clinician can develop strategies that promote the safe use of drugs during breastfeeding. The salient points in the use of drugs in breastfeeding are summarized below.

It is important that the following key points are considered when using of drugs during breastfeeding:

- Avoid drug use where this is possible.
- When drugs are needed, evaluate the infant dose and perform an individual risk–benefit analysis.
- For most drugs, a relative infant dose of < 10% of the maternal dose is safe.
- Choose drugs for which published data are available.
- Drugs with short half-lives, high protein binding or low oral bioavailability are preferred.
- Feeding towards the end of a dose interval may limit exposure for some drugs, while withholding periods are useful for others.
- Preterm or very young neonates are more susceptible to adverse effects from drugs in milk because their clearance mechanisms are not fully developed.
- When adverse effects are noted in very young infants, *in utero* exposure to drugs is a more likely cause than drug ingested in the milk.
- Many drugs are safe in breastfeeding mothers and the benefits of breastfeeding often outweigh the risks to the infant's wellbeing.
- A very small number of drugs are unsafe under any circumstances.

Index